Nutritional Management for COVID-19
&
Comorbidities

A handbook on right nutrition for
common & comorbid people

Swapan Banerjee, Suparna Das & Saroj Srivastava

Swapan Banerjee, Suparna Das, Saroj Srivastava

DEDICATION
The book is dedicated to those who lost their life
due to COVID-19 and its comorbidities

Swapan Banerjee, Suparna Das, Saroj Srivastava

CONTENT

1. INTRODUCTION

We can get good health by taking proper food. Good health is a result of adequate intake of the nutrient. Nutrition and fitness are interrelated; hence day by day, many diseases are affecting developing countries due to our faulty eating habits. Obesity is the most common disorder among them. According to the World Health Organisation, obesity and overweight are the unwanted fat deposition in the body that impairs our health. For adults, overweight is a BMI more than or equal to 22.9, and obesity >30. As per Asian value, 18.5-22.9 =normal range; overweight >23-24.9 ; pre obesity> 25-29.9; Obesity- 1st stage >30-39.9;obesity stage 2nd stage >40-49.9 ; and above 50 = morbid stage ,also called severe obesity. Obesity is not only found in adults but also in children and old aged people. As per the WHO data, the prevalence rate in 2016 was more than 2.0 billion adults, including eighteen years and older-aged who were overweight. Out of this population, approximately 648 million were obese, 40% of adults aged 18 years of age were overweight in 2017, and 13.9% were obese. The worldwide prevalence of obesity has nearly tripled between 1975 and 2016. [1] The primary reason for the occurrence of obesity is the imbalance between energy consumed and energy expenditure. The inclusion of energy-dense foods in which fat content is high and fiber content is low with insufficient or inadequate physical activity can lead to obesity. Urbanization, sedentary life, use of electronic gadgets reduces physical activity but increase the risk factors for our health [2]. Obesity can be prevented by proper diet and regular sufficient physical activities. It can cause health-related complications like respiratory problems, more prone to accidents, depression, and a lower lifespan if it is not treated. Obesity is considered a 'silent killer.' It can increase the chances of other diseases. Some of them are chronic and non-communicable also. Such as coronary heart disease, dyslipidemia, diabetes mellitus, gallbladder disease, hypertension, osteoarthritis, polycystic ovarian syndrome, thyroid disorders, fatty liver disease, some cancers

Part-I

2. CORONARY HEART DISEASE

Cardiovascular disease or Coronary heart disease is caused due to narrowing of the coronary arteries. So the blood flow is reduced, and the supply of oxygen, water, and nutrient are also reduced. This condition is also known as coronary artery disease (CAD). The narrowing of the coronary arteries happens due to the accumulation of cholesterol on the artery wall and forms plaque. Thereby the size of the lumen is reduced. This condition is known as atherosclerosis. Obese and people who are overweight have an excess cholesterol level in the blood. So they have more chance to develop atherosclerosis and Coronary heart disease also. When there is a reduced supply of oxygen-rich blood, nutrient, and water in the coronary artery, it commonly causes chest pain, known as angina pectoris. This is radiated down in the left arm.

The Heart attack results when the blood flow is not normal in the coronary artery, and as a result, a blood clot is formed. This condition is also known as myocardial infarction. World Health Organisation (WHO) has initiated 'Global Hearts' with the partners on the UN General Assembly's margins on 22nd Sept 2016 to beat against the global threat of cardiovascular disease, one of the leading causes of global death. [3]

PREVALENCE:

CHD is usually most common, along with obesity and overweight. It is one of the common causes of global death. According to WHO, 17.9 million people have died from cardiovascular disorders (CVD) by 2015-216. [4] Out of 7.4 million were killed due to coronary heart disease, and 6.7 million were died due to stroke. People with an unhealthy diet, less exercise, tobacco products, and alcohol consumption, hypertension (HTN), diabetes (DM), hyperlipidemia are at high risk of developing coronary heart disease [5].

AETIOLOGY:

Unhealthy Diet: High intake of calorie-dense foods, junk foods, and low intake of fiber-containing foods like vegetables, fruits for a prolonged period can lead to high blood cholesterol and also coronary heart disease.

Low physical activity: Physical inactivity with high-calorie intake can increase the risk of coronary heart disease. Regular physical activity can lower blood cholesterol, triglyceride and thereby helps to maintain blood pressure.

Obesity: Obesity and overweight are the predisposing factors for developing coronary heart disease. People with a high body mass index have a higher tendency to develop heart disease.

Lipid profile: People having a higher level of cholesterol (more than 200mg/100 ml blood), triglyceride, and low-density lipoprotein with lowered high-density lipoprotein in their blood have a greater tendency to develop atherosclerosis and as well as coronary heart disease.

Heredity: The hereditary tendency increased the risk of coronary heart diseases. It has been found that about 30 genes are involved in cardiovascular disease.

Age: the risk is higher in middle-aged people that are after the age of 5o years. Usually, young people are not suffering from coronary heart disease.

Sex: Men are at greater risk of developing coronary heart disease than women. But after menopause, women also tend to develop coronary heart disease.

Lifestyle: Those people who lead a sedentary lifestyle have a higher chance of developing heart disease. Alcohol intake and smoking, along with a sedentary lifestyle, can increase coronary heart disease rate, high blood pressure, and high blood cholesterol.

Hypertension: Hypertension is a predisposing factor that is usually associated with coronary heart disease. This is due to high blood pressure in hypertension, which increases the endothelial cell damage.

Diabetes mellitus: coronary heart disease and diabetes mellitus are associated with each other. This is because there are abnormalities in metabolism and insulin resistance in diabetes mellitus, enhancing cardiovascular disease rate.

FOOD SELECTION:

Foods to be excluded	Food to be taken moderately	Foods to be included
Red meat, sausages, organ meat, the fatty portion of meat, fatty fish, egg yolk, whole milk, cheese, ice cream, butter, ghee, mayonnaise, alcohol., table salt, canned food, salted chips, junk	Egg white, **a** simple sugar, honey, sugar syrup, cakes, chocolates, vegetable oils, margarine, nuts, sweetened beverages.	rice, wheat, bread, oats, puffed rice, rice flakes, green gram, Bengal gram, cowpea, lentils, and beans, **Roots and tubers,** lean meat, skimmed milk, yogurt, all fruits

foods, spicy foods, tobacco.		and fruit juices, fresh vegetables, tea, coffee, clear soups

DIET: Low-fat diet, which provides a low calorie, normal protein according to ideal body weight, is recommended for coronary heart disease. The carbohydrate (sugar) and sodium content of food in the daily diet should be modified. This is because diabetes and hypertension are associated with cardiovascular disease, and simple sugar and sodium content can increase blood sugar and blood pressure. [6]

FOOD TYPES SELECTION

Foodstuffs	Raw ingredients	
	Vegetarian	Non - vegetarian
Cereals (gm)	200	200
Pulses (gm)	60	40
Skimmed milk (ml)	100	100
Meat/fish (gm)	-	50
Green leafy vegetables (gm)	100	100
Other vegetables (gm)	100	100
Fruits (gm)	300	300
Sugar (gm)	40	40
Vegetable oil (gm)	50	50

The daily requirements of obese people with coronary heart disease are Calorie: 1800 kcal, Protein: 60 gm, Fat: 50 gm. The multivitamin tablets can be given to them as per advice from a physician. (This is a sample balanced diet; amount and result may vary from person to person).

3. DYSLIPIDEMIA

Dyslipidemia is a condition in which there is an abnormal level of cholesterol, triglycerides in the blood. Dyslipidemia is most common in developed countries as hyperlipidemia in which there is an elevation of mainly either cholesterol or triglycerides or both. It is a kind of lipid disorder. It is usually common in obese and overweight people due to a high-calorie diet and low physical activity. Lipids are carried in the blood by a transporter called lipoprotein formed by the conjugation of different lipid types: cholesterol, triglycerides, and phospholipids with the protein. Chylomicron, Very Low-Density Lipoprotein (VLDL), Intermediatory Density Lipoprotein (IDL), Low-Density Lipoprotein (LDL), High-Density Lipoprotein (HDL) are the different types of lipoprotein in our blood. The levels of lipoproteins are raised in dyslipidemia. The stories of other lipid parameters like cholesterol and triglycerides are also increased along with the raised level of lipoprotein. [7]

CLASSIFICATION:

The classification of lipid profile according to the National Cholesterol Education Programme ATP III report is as follows. . [8]

- LDL-Cholesterol level: Optimal: under 100 mg/dL, Near ideal/above optimal:100 to 129 mg/dL, Borderline high: 130 to 159 mg/dL, High: 160 to 189 mg/dL, Very high: more than 190 mg/dL.
- HDL C level: Low: under 40, high > 60.

- Fasting TGL level: Normal: under 150 mg/dL , Mild hypertriglyceridemia: 150 to 499 mg/dL, Moderate hypertriglyceridemia: 500 to 886 mg/dL. Very high or extreme hypertriglyceridemia > 886 mg/dL.

PREVALENCE:

Obesity and overweight harm, cholesterol, and triglycerides. Hyperlipidemia is associated with heredity, age, sex, lifestyle, high fat and calorie diet, etc. According to the World Health Organisation study, the global prevalence rate of elevated total cholesterol among adults was 39% in 2008. In developed countries, over 50% of adults with high economic levels have a high blood cholesterol level that is more than double of the lower-income countries according to the country's income level. [9]

AETIOLOGY:

Heredity: Genetic factor is a cause of familial hyperlipidemia. There is a familiar effect on hyperlipidemia.

Age: It is most common in people over 50 years of age. Young adults are not usually suffered from dyslipidemia. The risk factor is increased with age.

Sex: Male are more susceptible to develop dyslipidemia than females. But in the post-menopause phase, females also tend to develop hyperlipidemia.

Obesity: People with obesity and overweight have a greater chance of elevated levels of cholesterol, triglycerides, LDL cholesterol in their blood. A person who has a higher body mass index are more prone to develop hyperlipidemia.

Dietary habit: Intake of calorie-dense food, high fat, low fiber diet low physical activity for a prolonged period can increase cholesterol, triglycerides, LDL cholesterol in the blood and thereby increase chances to develop atherosclerosis and other heart diseases.

Lifestyle: A sedentary lifestyle that is a low physical activity with an excess of tobacco and alcohol can increase the risk of developing hyperlipidemia.

Others: Diabetes, hypothyroidism, renal disease, liver disease, and some other drugs like glucocorticoids, oral contraceptives can impair lipid metabolism, leading to an increased cholesterol level, triglycerides, LDL cholesterol blood. Mainly these are secondary causes of dyslipidemia.

FOOD SELECTION:

Foods to be excluded	Food to be taken moderately	Foods to be included
Red meat, sausages, organ meat, the fatty portion of meat, fatty fish, egg yolk, whole milk, cheese, ice cream, butter, ghee, alcohol, table salt, canned food, salted chips, junk foods, spicy foods, tobacco.	Egg white, **a** simple sugar, honey, sugar syrup, cakes, chocolates, vegetable oils, margarine, nuts, sweetened beverages.	rice, wheat, bread, oats, puffed rice, rice flakes, green gram, Bengal gram, cowpea, lentils and beans, lean meat, skimmed milk, yogurt, all fruits and fruit juices, fresh vegetables, tea, coffee, clear soups

DIET: A low-fat diet that provides normal calorie normal protein according to ideal body weight is recommended for dyslipidemia. Sodium and simple sugar should be restricted if hypertension and diabetes mellitus is present, respectively. Restriction of foods that rich in cholesterol should be done. A patient having hyperlipidemia should include fiber-containing food in his daily diet. The daily requirements of obese people with dyslipidemia are Calorie: 1600 kcal, Protein: 60 gm, Fat: 25 gm [10]

FOOD TYPES SELECTION:

Foodstuffs	Raw ingredients	
	Vegetarian	Non - vegetarian
Cereals (gm)	200	200
Pulses (gm)	80	60
Skimmed milk (ml)	700	700
Meat/fish (gm)	-	75
Green leafy vegetables (gm)	100	100
Other vegetables (gm)	100	100
Fruits (gm)	100	100
Sugar (gm)	30	30
Vegetable oil (gm)	25	25

The multivitamin tablet can also be given to them after medical advice from a physician. (This is a sample balanced diet; amount and result may vary from person to person).

4. DIABETES MELLITUS

Diabetes mellitus is a chronic metabolic disorder in which there is an increased blood sugar level for a prolonged period, characterized by the body's inability or decreased ability to utilize glucose properly. There are faulty carbohydrate metabolism and improper metabolism of protein and fat, and damaging water and electrolyte balance. In severe infections, it also affects the vascular system of the kidney, heart, eye, brain, etc. In India, a person with a high blood sugar level is called 'Madhumeha' (hyperglycemia). Obese or overweight people have a higher chance of developing diabetes mellitus. Obesity can cause impaired insulin uptake by the receptors of the target, which may lead to hyperglycemia. [11]

The common symptoms are such as Polyuria (excessive urination), Polydipsia (increased thirst), Dry mouth, Polyphagia (increased hunger), Fatigue, weight loss, delay in wound healing, water, and electrolyte imbalance, etc.

According to the American Diabetic Association, the diagnostic criteria for diabetes mellitus are as follows:

Fasting Plasma Glucose level should be below or standard 126 (7.0). The test should be acted in a research facility by utilizing the NGSP strategy, affirmed and normalized by the DCCT test. A patient with reasonable indications for hyperglycemic emergency hyperglycemia or an irregular plasma glucose level $\geq$of 200 milligrams per Decilitre (11.1 Milimoles per Liter) [12].

TYPE: Diabetes mellitus can be of different types. Some common forms among them are listed below, such as Type-1, also called Insulin Dependent Diabetes Mellitus (IDDM), Type II DM, i.e., Non-Insulin Dependent Diabetes Mellitus (NIDDM), Maturity Onset Diabetes of the Young (MODY), Gestational Diabetes

Mellitus, Malnutrition Related Diabetes Mellitus (MRDM). There are some other types of diabetes mellitus, such as Genetic defects in β-cell function, Genetic defects in insulin action, Fibro Calculus, Pancreatic Diabetes (FCPD), Chronic pancreatic diabetes, Endocrinopathies.

PREVALENCE:

Insulin-dependent diabetes mellitus (type I) diabetes is less in numbers but often seen at a young age or in children. This is why it is also called juvenile diabetes, and sometimes undernourished children develop IDDM [13]. Type II diabetes mellitus is mainly found in an adult person. Obese and overweight people with a lack of exercise are more prevalent to develop diabetes mellitus type II than ordinary people. Sedentary lifestyle-based people live in developed countries highly susceptible to non-insulin-dependent diabetes mellitus (type II), which is also very common worldwide at old age. [14] According to the World Health Organisation, the number of people with diabetes has risen from 108 million in 1980 to 422 million in 2014. The global prevalence of diabetes among adults over 18 years of age increased from 4.7% in 1980 to 8.5% in 2014. [15]

Here we briefly discuss Type I / Insulin-dependent diabetes mellitus (IDDM) and Type II / Non-insulin-dependent diabetes mellitus (NIDDM).

5. DIABETES MELLITUS (TYPE I)

Insulin-dependent diabetes mellitus (IDDM) is a type of diabetes mellitus. It is characterized by high blood sugar levels in the body. This condition is found due to small or inadequate or no insulin hormone production from the β-cells of islets of Langerhans of the pancreas. It is also known as 'Juvenile onset Diabetes.' Acidosis in this condition is usually common. [16]

AETIOLOGY:

Genetics: It involves a different type of genes. The hereditary tendency can increase the chances of the development of type I diabetes mellitus mostly. Human Lymphocyte Antigen is mainly responsible for this occurrence.

Environment: Along with hereditary factors environment can also enhance the risk of type I diabetes mellitus.

Virus infection: People with type I diabetes mellitus sometimes suffer from Coxsackie or any other virus infection. Study reveals that this Coxsackie infection can trigger the autoimmune response, and due to this, our immune system attacks the infected cell and the β-cell of the pancreas. Thus insulin secretion from the β-cell of the pancreas is hampered.

Immunity: Insulin-dependent diabetes mellitus (type I) is an autoimmune disease and is also associated with a different kind of autoimmune disorder. [17]

Stress: Any type of acute stress from physical injury, trauma, accident, surgery can lead to a variety I diabetes mellitus. Stress can lead to the secretion of any catabolic hormone associated with Insulin-dependent diabetes mellitus.

Diet: Those young children who take a fat-rich and low fiber diet tend to develop this disorder. Diets rich in gluten increase intestinal permeability and allow foreign particles' entrance that leads to infection in the body, associated with type- I diabetes Mellitus.

6. DIABETES MELLITUS (TYPE II)

Non-Insulin dependent diabetes mellitus (NIDDM) is another type of diabetes mellitus that lasts forever. It is characterized by high blood sugar in the body due to insulin resistance and a relative lack of insulin. [18] It is found to develop slowly and usually more stable and milder than type I. In this condition, an adequate amount of insulin may be secreted, but their action is hampered.

AETIOLOGY:

Genetics: Genetic factors play a more critical role in developing NIDDM than IDDM. People of developing countries like India have a genetic risk of developing diabetes. Sometimes there is the mutation of the Glucokinase gene, which is associated with maturity-onset diabetes mellitus.

Age: Diabetes is usually occurring in any period of life, but the type II diabetes mellitus is more common in elder or mild aged people.

Sex: Males and females both have an equal risk of developing this type of diabetes mellitus.

Obesity: Obesity is another crucial cause of developing diabetes mellitus. People of a sedentary lifestyle, along with low physical activity and high fat and soft fiber-rich diet, have greater chances of this type of diabetes mellitus.

Insulin resistance: Insulin resistance is not the ability to maintain the glucose level in the blood by the body in the presence of an average level of insulin that is linked with type II diabetes mellitus and also with obesity.

Pregnancy: High blood sugar level in pregnancy is referred to as 'gestational diabetes.' It is due to changes in hormonal levels in pregnancy. But it is usually disappeared after the delivery, but if it is continued, then proper treatment should be required. [19]

Virus infection: Different kind of virus infection such as chickenpox, measles, and mumps can lower immunity and also helps in some autoimmune reaction, which can destroy the β-cells of the pancreas that secretes insulin that indirectly associated with this type of diabetes.

Stress: Stress releases some adrenaline and nor-adrenaline hormone, which act as the opposite function of insulin, leading to type II diabetes mellitus.

FOOD SELECTION:

Foods to be excluded	Food to be taken moderately	Foods to be included
simple sugar, jaggery, molasses, honey, sugar syrup, cakes, chocolates, red meat, a fatty portion of meat, sausages, fatty fish, egg yolk.\, whole milk, cheese, butter, ghee, mayonnaise, sweetened beverages, table salt, canned food, salted chips, junk foods	rice, wheat, bread, oats, puffed rice, rice flakes, green gram, Bengal gram, cowpea, lentils and beans, Roots, lean meat, channa, paneer, vegetable oils, butter, margarine, nuts	egg white, skimmed milk, yogurt, all fruits and fruit juices except banana, mango, litchi, jackfruit, fresh vegetables, tea, coffee, clear soups, spices

DIET: Along with medicine and insulin therapy, diet is a preventive factor for diabetes mellitus. Food intake should be helpful for adequate insulin secretion in Insulin-dependent diabetes mellitus (IDDM). Usually, the diet includes complex saccharides, high dietary fiber, low fat, moderate protein, sufficient vitamins, and minerals with regular physical activity is highly recommended for diabetic patients. The daily requirements of obese people with Diabetes mellitus are Calorie: 1200 kcal, Protein: 45 gm, Fat: 30 gm, Carbohydrate: 188 gm. [20]

FOOD TYPES SELECTION:

Foodstuffs	Raw ingredients	
	Vegetarian	Non - vegetarian
Cereals (gm)	175	200
Pulses (gm)	40	20
Skimmed milk (ml)	300	150
Meat/fish (gm)	-	70
Green leafy vegetables (gm)	100	100
Other vegetables (gm)	100	100
Fruits (gm)	100	100
Oil (gm)	30	50

(This is a sample plan, so the quantity and result may vary from person to person).

7. HYPERTENSION

According to the World Health Organisation, 'Hypertension, also known as high or raised blood pressure, is a condition in which the blood vessels have persistently raised pressure.' [21] Blood elevates lateral pressure in the artery while passing through the arteries in the heart. The state is referred to as blood pressure. The average systolic blood pressure is 120 mmHg, and diastolic blood pressure (DBP) is 80 mm Hg in adults. Hypertension is a condition in which systolic blood pressure (SBP) exceeds 160 mm Hg and diastolic blood pressure exceeds 95 mm Hg. Body weights have a direct effect on hypertension. It is observed that hypertension is most common in overweight and obese people. Hypertension increases due to increasing body mass index (BMI) than the normal range. [22]

The study reveals that the blood pressures of the participants were measured. Among them, those who had not any history of hypertension were categorized as normal blood pressure (<120/80 mm Hg), elevated Blood pressure (120–129/<80 mm Hg), hypertension stage I (130–139/80–89 mm Hg), and hypertension stage II (≥140/90 mm Hg) and those participants with a history of hypertension were classified as they were treated and strictly controlled hypertension (<130/80 mm Hg after using antihypertensive medicine), treated and controlled hypertension (130–139/80–89 mm Hg after using antihypertensive medication), treated but uncontrolled hypertension (≥140/90 mm Hg after using antihypertensive medicine), and not treated hypertension (after not using antihypertensive medication). [23]

PREVALENCE:

The prevalence rate of hypertension is higher in males as compared to women. The prevalence of hypertension is increased with age.

Urban people have more chances to develop hypertension than people living in rural areas. Hypertension is a common comorbidity associated with diabetes, obesity, and other lifestyle disorders among older persons, mainly in urban areas. The sedentary worker who has less physical activity become overweight and also develop hypertension as compared to others. Lifestyle, stress, dietary habit, workload also affect the occurrences of hypertension. [24]. WHO estimates that 1.56 billion adults will be living with hypertension in the year 2025. [25]

AETIOLOGY:

Age: Hypertension is more common in aged people. Workload, stress is increased with age. Therefore the chance of occurrence of hypertension is high in the older individual. But now day adolescence and even young adults have hypertension.

Gender: Male has a higher chance of developing hypertension than women. But after menopause, the female also has an increased opportunity to develop hypertension. [26]

Heredity: It is believed that heredity is a predisposing factor of hypertension.

Lifestyle: A person with a sedentary lifestyle with low physical activity, smoking, tobacco intake, alcohol intake has a higher chance of developing hypertension.

Hormone: Hormones like aldosterone, rennin, angiotensin regulate blood pressure along with water and electrolyte balance. Thus it is related to hypertension. Other hormones like adrenaline, nor-adrenaline, cortisone, which are secreted due to stress, can lead to hypertension due to the narrowing of blood vessels. [27]

Obesity: Obesity is another essential predisposing factor of hypertension. An increase in body weight may increase the risk of hypertension. Obesity is a responsible factor in developing any cardiovascular disease which is directly associated with hypertension. [28]

Other physiological conditions: Along with cardiovascular diseases, renal disease, hyperthyroidism, diabetes, nervous system disorder can also aggravate the chances to develop hypertension.

FOOD SELECTION:

Foods to be excluded	Food to be taken moderately	Foods to be included
Red meat, the fatty portion of meat, fatty fish, egg yolk, whole milk, cheese, ice cream, butter, ghee, mayonnaise, honey, sugar syrup, cakes, chocolates, sweetened beverages, alcohol, table salt, canned food, salted chips, junk foods, tobacco.	Egg white, **a** simple sugar, vegetable oil, margarine, nuts, channa, paneer.	rice, wheat, bread, oats, puffed rice, rice flakes, green gram, Bengal gram, cowpea, lentils and beans, **Roots and tubers,** lean meat, skimmed milk, yogurt, all fruits and fruit juices, fresh vegetables, tea, coffee, clear soups, spices

DIET: Low sodium, a low fat, low-calorie diet which contains normal protein, is recommended for people having hypertension. In severe hypertension, sometimes protein is moderated because protein foods are rich in sodium. [29] DASH (Dietary approach to stop hypertension) diet can be followed to treat high blood pressure. The patient can take whole grain cereals, lean meat, vegetables, fruit, dairy products, etc. The daily requirements of obese people with hypertension are Calorie: 1800 kcal, Protein: 60 gm, Fat: 30 gm. [29] [30]

FOOD TYPES SELECTION

Foodstuffs	Raw ingredients	
	Vegetarian	Non - vegetarian
Cereals (gm)	200	200
Pulses (gm)	60	40
Skimmed milk (ml)	800	800
Meat/fish (gm)	-	50
Green leafy vegetables (gm)	100	100
Other vegetables (gm)	100	100
Fruits (gm)	200	200
Sugar (gm)	30	30
Vegetable oil (gm)	30	30

Medication: the multivitamin tablet can also be given to them after medical advice from the physician.

(This is a sample plan, so the amount and result may vary from person to person).

8. GALLBLADDER DISEASE

The gallbladder is a pear-shaped little sac type organ attached to the right side of the liver. Bile is formed in the liver and stored in the gallbladder. The gallbladder's primary role in our body is to keep and concentrate bile from the liver. Gallbladder contracts and releases bile through a tube, which is called the common bile duct. This tube connects our gallbladder and liver to the small intestine. When food has come into the small intestine from the stomach during digestion, the common bile duct carries bile to the small intestine to help in this process. This bile contains bile pigments (bilirubin and biliverdin), bile salts (sodium glycocholate and sodium taurocholate), cholesterol, fat, and water. Obese people have a higher chance of developing gallbladder disease. Obesity with high blood cholesterol can aggravate the condition [31-38].

There are many disorders found in the gallbladder. The most common diseases of the gallbladder are as follows:

Cholelithiasis: Gallbladder stone is also known as cholelithiasis. It is an asymptomatic condition. Patients usually feel pain after eating. There are a few kinds of gallstones. These are as follows -

Cholesterol stone: This type of stone is usually tiny, challenging, and greenish-yellow in color. It is formed due to excess cholesterol deposition. This cholesterol is then saturated and crystallized in the gallbladder.

Pigmented stone: This type of stone is usually small and dark in color. It is made up of bile pigments (bilirubin and biliverdin) and formed due to hemolysis.

Mixed stone: This type of stone usually contain cholesterol, calcium salt, bile pigments (bilirubin and other bile pigments).

Biliary sludge: It is a result of complications due to intravenous feeding.

1. **Choledocholithiasis:** When the stone is present in the bile duct, this condition is referred to as choledocholithiasis. It obstructs the biliary duct that leads to pain.
2. **Cholecystitis:** When there is inflammation in the gallbladder, it is known as cholecystitis. It is usually found due to gallstones in the bile duct. This stone can cause the backflow of bile, leading to infection on the wall of the gallbladder. It can be of two types. These are as follows -

Acute cholecystitis: 80% of acute cholecystitis is caused by a gallstone. Sometimes it is also caused by without stones

Chronic cholecystitis: chronic cholecystitis is caused due to repeated occurrences of gallstones.

PREVALENCE: [38-42]

1. The prevalence rate of gallbladder disease is higher in obese people with a sedentary lifestyle and high blood cholesterol.
2. According to the World Gastroenterology Organisation, more than 85 % of gallstones are cholesterol stones in developed countries.
3. Studies reveal that about 10 – 15% of gallstone patients have the chances of recurrences of the gallbladder and common bile duct stones.

AETIOLOGY: [42-47]

Obesity: It is one of the most significant risk factors for gallbladder disease. Obesity with high blood cholesterol can raise the percentage of cholesterol in the bile. So it can cause cholesterol gallstone.

Age: It is not common in young people. It is usually found in old aged people.

Sex: Females have a greater tendency to develop gallbladder disease. It may be due to fat deposition in their body, which is regulated by the female sex hormone that is estrogen.

Lifestyle: The chance of developing gallbladder disease is increased with the sedentary lifestyle. High-calorie intake with low or absence of regular physical activity can increase the risk factor.

Heredity: Family history is one of the predisposing factors of gallbladder stones.

Others: some diseases like diabetes mellitus, inflammatory disease, and some drugs like oral contraceptives can also aggravate this condition.

FOOD SELECTION: [44-48]

FOODS TO BE EXCLUDED	FOOD TO BE TAKEN MODERATELY	FOODS TO BE INCLUDED

MEAT: red meat, a fatty portion of meat FISH: Fatty fish EGG: egg yolk MILK AND MILK PRODUCTS: whole milk, ice cream, mayonnaise NUTS AND OIL: butter, ghee, cheese, nuts SUGAR: sweets FRUITS: dried fruits BEVERAGES: thick soup, alcohol. OTHERS: table salt, canned food, salted chips, junk foods, fried food, pickle, condiments, tobacco.	EGG: egg white (if no problem indigestion) OIL: vegetable oil, margarine MEAT: Lean meat	CEREAL: rice, wheat, bread, oats, puffed rice, rice flakes. PULSES: green gram, Bengal gram, cowpea, lentils, and beans ROOTS AND TUBERS FISH AND FISH OIL MILK AND MILK PRODUCTS: Skimmed Milk, yogurt, channa, paneer. SUGAR: Honey, jaggery FRUITS: all fruits and fruit juices VEGETABLES: fresh vegetables BEVERAGES: tea, coffee, clear soups OTHERS: spices, jam, jelly

DIET:

Low fat, low-calorie, average protein diet that contains normal carbohydrate is recommended for people with gallbladder disorders. But simple carbohydrate intake should be reduced, and fiber must be present in the daily diet. Vitamins, minerals supplementation may be needed. High fluid intake is also suggested.

The daily requirements of obese people with gall bladder disease are as follows:

1. Calorie: 1200 - 1400 kcal.
2. Protein: 70gm.
3. Fat: 15gm.

FOOD TYPES SELECTION:

FOODSTUFFS	RAW INGREDIENTS	
	VEGETARIAN	NON-VEGETARIAN
CEREALS (gm)	175	175
PULSES (gm)	75	60
SKIMMED MILK (ml)	800	800
MEAT/FISH (gm)	-	75
GREEN LEAFY VEGETABLES (gm)	100	100
OTHER VEGETABLES (gm)	100	100
FRUITS (gm)	100	100
SUGAR (gm)	10	10
VEGETABLE OIL (gm)	15	15

The multivitamin tablet can also be given to them after medical advice from a physician. (This is a sample plan; so, the quantity and responses are person wise variable).

9. OSTEOARTHRITIS

Osteoarthritis is a common form of arthritis. It is a degenerative disorder of joints. It is a chronic disease that is found due to the breakdown of the joint cartilage.

In normal condition, the ends of bones in joints are covered by cartilage, a firm, rubbery and slippery tissue. A healthy Cartilage provides smoothness, cushioning effect between the bones and absorbs the shocks during movement. But in osteoarthritis, this joint cartilage is broken down and can cause joint pain. When the joint cartilage is broken, a bone comes in contact with another bone and then rubs together. This rubbing of bones is when permanent, it can cause damage to the bone joint. Osteoarthritis can be found in any joint of the body but commonly affects the knees, spine, neck, hips, and fingers' joints.

Osteoarthritis is also known as "wear and tear" of joints. It involves not only joint cartilage but also bone, ligament, and joint linings. Breakdown of the joint cartilage means losing the joints' protection layer in the body [49-52].

TYPES: Based on the diagnosis, osteoarthritis can be classified into two types. These are the following:

Primary Osteoarthritis: It is mainly connected with aging. This type of osteoarthritis is mostly found in aged people whose age is above 55 years. This type of osteoarthritis is primarily developed in certain joints. So this type can be again subdivided based on the affected sites like knee osteoarthritis, hip osteoarthritis, Trapeziometacarpal osteoarthritis in hands, wrist osteoarthritis.

Secondary osteoarthritis: This type of osteoarthritis is mainly found in young people. Some conditions like trauma, infection, metabolic problem, gout, rheumatoid arthritis can aggravate this condition. Primarily it is developed due to changes in the environment of the cartilage. [53]

SYMPTOMS: The symptoms of osteoarthritis are usually developed slowly, and over time the condition becomes worse. It includes pain, stiffness, bone spurs, loss of flexibility, tenderness, grating sensation, loss of ability, sometimes joints may be filled with fluid.

PREVALENCE:

According to the World Health Organisation (WHO), 18.0% of women and 9.6% of men have symptomatic osteoarthritis whose age is over 60. Among them, 80% have the limitation in movement, and 25% have the problem performing their daily life activities.

In India, the prevalence rate of osteoarthritis is from 22 to 39%.

AETIOLOGY: [54]

Age: Osteoarthritis is directly associated with age. It is increased with age over time.

Sex: Men, Women both are at risk of developing osteoarthritis. But women have higher chances of getting this.

Obesity: Obesity and overweight contribute extra load, especially on the hip and knees. Weight-bearing for several days can cause the breakdown of joint cartilages of the body. Excess calorie intake with low fibers, vitamins, and minerals can be increased the rate of osteoarthritis.

Sedentary lifestyle: Physically low activity or inactivity can also weaker the muscle and tendons present in joints' surroundings.

Heredity: Family history is a predisposing factor for osteoarthritis. Some people have a hereditary tendency to develop osteoarthritis.

Bone deformities: some people have inborn defective cartilage that can increase the condition to develop osteoarthritis.

Joint injuries: Sometimes, people are facing some joint injuries from any accidents, playing sports. That can lead to osteoarthritis.

Occupational activity: Some occupations involve stress on joints repetitively; slowly, it can lead to osteoarthritis.

Other conditions: Neuromuscular diseases, neuropathy, rheumatoid arthritis, gout can cause extra stress and inflammation on the joint that can worsen the situation.

FOOD SELECTION: [52-54]

FOODS TO BE EXCLUDED	FOOD TO BE TAKEN MODERATELY	FOODS TO BE INCLUDED

MEAT: red meat, the fatty portion of meat FISH: Fatty fish EGG: egg yolk MILK AND MILK PRODUCTS: whole milk, ice cream, mayonnaise NUTS AND OIL: butter, ghee, cheese, nuts SUGAR: sweets FRUITS: dried fruits BEVERAGES: thick soup, alcohol. OTHERS: table salt, canned food, salted chips, junk foods, fried food, pickle, condiments, tobacco.	EGG: egg white (if no problem indigestion) OIL: vegetable oil, margarine MEAT: Lean meat	CEREAL: rice, wheat, bread, oats, puffed rice, rice flakes. PULSES: green gram, Bengal gram, cowpea, lentils, and beans ROOTS AND TUBERS MILK AND MILK PRODUCTS: Skimmed Milk, yogurt, channa, paneer. SUGAR: Honey, jaggery FRUITS: all fruits and fruit juices VEGETABLES: fresh vegetables BEVERAGES: tea, coffee, clear soups OTHERS: spices, jam, jelly

DIET:

Low fat, low-calorie, average protein diet that contains normal carbohydrate, vitamins, and minerals are recommended for people suffering from osteoarthritis. But carbohydrates should be taken in complex form, and fiber must be present in the daily diet. Vitamins, minerals supplementation could be taken but after consultation with a doctor and dietician.

The daily requirements of obese people with osteoarthritis are as follows:

1. Calorie: 1400 - 1600 kcal.

2. Protein: 70 gm.
3. Fat: 15, gm.
4. Calcium: 2000 IU

FOOD TYPES SELECTION:

FOODSTUFFS	RAW INGREDIENTS	
	VEGETARIAN	NON - VEGETARIAN
CEREALS (gm)	200	200
PULSES (gm)	80	40
SKIMMED MILK (ml)	1000	1000
MEAT/FISH (gm)	-	75
GREEN LEAFY VEGETABLES (gm)	100	100
OTHER VEGETABLES (gm)	100	100
FRUITS (gm)	100	100
SUGAR (gm)	25	25
VEGETABLE OIL (gm)	15	15

Supplementation: Calcium supplements can also be given to them after medical advice from the physician. Other medications - As per physician's advice or prescriptions based on age, BMI, activities, etc.

10. POLYCYSTIC OVARIAN SYNDROME

Polycystic ovarian syndrome is also known as polycystic ovarian disease. It is a condition in which there is an imbalance between female sex hormones and estrogen and progesterone.

Usually, female ovaries produce female sex hormones that are estrogen and progesterone and a few amounts of male sex hormone that is testosterone (well-known primary androgen). Polycystic ovarian syndrome is caused by an imbalance of all of these sex hormones.

These hormones help to regulate the normal ovulation cycle. The ovulation cycle is one in which one or more mature eggs are released from the female ovaries in each menstrual cycle every month. These eggs are present in the ovarian follicle, which is a sac-like part of the ovaries. In Polycystic ovarian syndrome, the production of androgen hormone, a male sex hormone, is slightly elevated than the female body's average level. Therefore, menstrual cycles become irregular for a prolonged period, and for this, the eggs cannot mature in the ovarian follicle and are not released from the ovaries. These eggs remain present in the ovarian follicle. These can come from many (poly) tiny cysts in the female ovaries. Hence it is named polycystic ovarian disease.

It is a lifestyle disorder. The actual treatment of PCOS is not discovered. But losing bodyweight, proper diet, and regular exercise can reduce the complication [55].

TYPES:

SYMPTOMS: Polycystic ovarian syndrome is characterized by irregular menstruation cycle, fertility problem while getting pregnant, weight gain, acne, excess body and facial hair, depression. It is also increased the risk of heart disease, high blood pressure, diabetes, uterine cancer.

PREVALENCE:

Polycystic ovarian syndrome is found in the reproductive age group, especially between 18 and 45.

It usually affects 2 – 20% of women in their reproductive age group. * According to the US Department of Health and Human Services, 5 million women already have the polycystic ovarian syndrome.

AETIOLOGY:

The exact cause of the polycystic ovarian syndrome is not known till now. But there may be some following factors that increase the risk of this disorder.

Heredity: Genetics is a predisposing factor for polycystic ovarian syndrome. Some women in their reproductive age group develop PCOS whose mother or sister have also have this disorder.

Hormonal imbalance: Abnormal elevation of male sex hormone, androgen hormone, and decreased secretion of female sex hormone estrogen can cause difficulties in ovulation. Hence egg is not released with menstruation every month.

Obesity: Some women having excess body weight. It leads to an irregular menstruation cycle. Hence there is difficulty in getting pregnant.

Dietary habits: Irregular nutritional patterns, skipping meals can cause low nutritional status. Intake of the high-calorie diet with the absence or insufficient amount of fiber, vitamins, and minerals can increase the body weight, which indirectly enhances the risk of developing the polycystic ovarian syndrome.

Lifestyle: Sedentary lifestyle with low physical activity, excess alcohol intake, and smoking can hamper the function of the reproductive organs.

Others: Stressful life, anxiety, tension can also cause hormonal imbalance in the reproductive age group of women [58].

FOOD SELECTION: [56-57]

FOODS TO BE EXCLUDED	FOOD TO BE TAKEN MODERATELY	FOODS TO BE INCLUDED

MEAT: red meat, the fatty portion of meat FISH: Fatty fish. EGG: egg yolk MILK AND MILK PRODUCTS: whole milk, ice cream, mayonnaise NUTS AND OIL: butter, ghee, cheese, nuts SUGAR: sweets FRUITS: dried fruits BEVERAGES: thick soup, alcohol. OTHERS: table salt, canned food, salted chips, junk foods, fried food, pickle, condiments, tobacco.	EGG: egg white (if no problem indigestion) OIL: vegetable oil, margarine MEAT: Lean meat	CEREAL: rice, wheat, bread, oats, puffed rice, rice flakes. PULSES: green gram, Bengal gram, cowpea, lentils, and beans ROOTS AND TUBERS MILK AND MILK PRODUCTS: Skimmed Milk, yogurt, channa, paneer. SUGAR: Honey, jaggery FRUITS: all fruits and fruit juices VEGETABLES: fresh vegetables BEVERAGES: tea, coffee, clear soups OTHERS: spices, jam, jelly

DIET:

A regular and healthy diet containing low-fat, low-calorie, ordinary protein, normal carbohydrate, vitamins, and minerals are recommended for people suffering from osteoarthritis. Fiber must be present in the daily diet.

The daily requirements of obese people with polycystic ovarian disease are as follows:

1. Calorie: 1400 kcal.
2. Protein: 60, gm.
3. Fat: 20, gm.

FOOD TYPES SELECTION :

FOODSTUFFS	RAW INGREDIENTS	
	VEGETARIAN	NON - VEGETARIAN
CEREALS (gm)	175	200
PULSES (gm)	80	60
SKIMMED MILK (ml)	500	300
MEAT/FISH (gm)	-	75
GREEN LEAFY VEGETABLES (gm)	100	100
OTHER VEGETABLES (gm)	100	100
FRUITS (gm)	100	100
SUGAR (gm)	25	25
VEGETABLE OIL (gm)	20	20

[This is a sample plan so that results may vary per person].

11.THYROID DISORDERS

Thyroid disorders are a condition that can affect the thyroid gland and, thereby, its function. The thyroid gland is an endocrine gland situated in the front of the neck, below Adam's apple. It is a butterfly-shaped gland; consists of two lobes that are connected by the isthmus. Thyroid gland secret essential hormones are triiodothyronine (T3) and Thyroxine (T4) with tyrosine and iodine. These hormones regulate most of the metabolism in the body, including protein synthesis. Hypothyroidism is also associated with faulty fat metabolism and even with weight gain.

The function of the thyroid gland is regulated by a mechanism known as the feedback mechanism. When there is a lower secretion of thyroid hormones, the brain helps produce a thyrotropin-releasing hormone (TRH). It causes the secretion of thyroid-stimulating hormone (TSH) by the posterior pituitary. This thyroid-stimulating hormone then stimulates the thyroid gland to secrete more thyroxine hormone [59-60].

Genetic Factors: Various types of thyroid disorders are also responsible due to genetic factors. Therefore, there are some tests available to confirm genetic matters.

TYPES:

There are different types of thyroid disorders. Those are described as follow-

TYPE	DESCRIPTION
Hypothyroidism	It is a condition when there is an inadequate release of thyroid hormones by the thyroid gland.
Hyperthyroidism	It is a condition when there is the overproduction of thyroid hormones by the thyroid gland.
Goiter	This condition is described as the abnormal enlargement of the butterfly-shaped thyroid gland

Thyroid nodules	These nodules are lumps like masses in the thyroid gland. A cyst, the tumor can cause it.
Thyroiditis	This condition is usually described as an inflammation of the thyroid gland.
Thyroid cancer	There is cancer within the thyroid gland. It may be due to a cancerous tumor.

SYMPTOMS:

The symptoms are varying with the type of thyroid disorders. The most common symptoms of hypothyroidism and hyperthyroidism

Hypothyroidism - Weight gain, depression, tiredness, constipation, cold sensation, memory difficulties, muscle and joint pain, slow heart rate.

Hyperthyroidism- Weight loss, diarrhea, sensitivity to hot temperature, insomnia, increased sweating, fast heart rate, nervousness [61].

PREVALENCE:

According to the American Association of Clinical Endocrinologists, thyroid disorders are more common in women.

Out of 10, 8 patients are women having thyroid diseases. The prevalence rates are high among pregnant women and people having overweight.

AETIOLOGY: [61-62]

Hypothyroidism is caused by Graves' disease, Toxic adenomas, Subacute thyroiditis, malfunction of the pituitary gland, and hyperthyroidism is caused by Hashimoto's disease, thyroid gland removal, drugs like lithium, excess amount of iodine intake. Some common causes of thyroid problems are as follows -

Heredity: genetics is the most common cause of both hypothyroidism and hyperthyroidism.

Sex: Hypothyroidism can be found among both males and females. But it is most common in women, and even some symptoms also vary between genders.

Age: Thyroid disorder is commonly found among older people. Hypothyroidism is usually common in older people above 50 years of age.

Dietary Habit: Diet deficiency in iodine can cause insufficient production of hypothyroidism, and it may lead to goiter. Excess consumption of tea, coffee can decrease the iodine absorption from the daily diet.

Obesity and Lifestyle: There is a greater chance of increased thyroid-stimulating hormone with increased body weight above the normal. A sedentary lifestyle with stress, anxiety, and tobacco and alcohol use can increase the risk of thyroid disorders [63].

 Others: Autoimmune diseases, diabetes, heart diseases are also associated with thyroid disorders [64].

FOOD SELECTION:

FOODS TO BE EXCLUDED	FOOD TO BE TAKEN MODERATELY	FOODS TO BE INCLUDED
Cyanogenic foods: Kernel foods, Almonds, Apricots, Cherries, Peaches, plant seeds, Cassava, including some more stems, contain lectin. **Goitrogenic:** Cabbage, kale, Cassava, Cauliflower, Soy, Spinach, Rapeseed, Mustard, Broccoli, Millets, Peanuts, Sweet potatoes, Turnip, Strawberries, Pear, Peaches. **Thiocyanate:** Cigarette smoke. **Cruciferous plants:** cabbage, cauliflower, mustard (seeds and leaves), turnip, radish, brussels sprouts. **Genistein, Glycitein & Daidzein** (Phytoestrogen): Isoflavone found in Soy, Coffee, fava beans. **Resveratrol-phytoalexin-** Dark chocolate, blueberries, cranberries, peanuts, pistachios, grapes, red	**Greens**: produced from the ground where pesticides, herbicides are often used. **Fruits** –Grapefruits and grapefruit juices, all sweet artificial canned foods and fruits.	**Iodine** from table salt within 5 gm-10gm per day. Some more quantity of an **onion, garlic, ginger.** As a supplement, Aloe vera juice is helpful. Some studies talk about drum stick is helpful [65].

wine. Caffeine – Coffee may impair thyroid health. **Synthetic/ halogenated flavonoid** Tea, Citrus Fruit, Citrus Fruit Juices, Berries, Red Wine, Apples, Legumes.		

The average energy for hypothyroidism can be 1200-1600kcal/day.

1. Calorie: 1400 kcal.
2. Protein: 60, gm.
3. Fat: 20, gm.

FOOD TYPES SELECTION:

FOODSTUFFS	RAW INGREDIENTS	
	VEGETARIAN	NON - VEGETARIAN
CEREALS (gm)	180	200
PULSES (gm)	70	70
SKIMMED MILK (ml)	500	300
MEAT/FISH (gm)	-	75-100gm

GREEN LEAFY VEGETABLES (gm)	200	100
OTHER VEGETABLES (gm)	100	-
FRUITS (gm)	200	200
SUGAR (gm)	20	20
VEGETABLE OIL (gm)	30	30

Note:

*

*

*

*

*

*

*

*

*

*

*

*

*

*

*

*

*

Part-II- COVID -19

*

*

*

*

*

*

*

12. Corona Virus (COVID-19) -Introduction

Corona Virus, i.e., Covid-19, is an infectious condition that spreads from one person to another through droplets when these droplets get into your eyes, nose, and mouth. The organs associated are mostly upper (URTI) respiratory tract organs such as the nose, larynx, throat, and parts of the lungs. Novel Corona Virus was identified first in China at Wuhan province in December 2019. Coronavirus shows very much infectious for the comorbid patients identified with a low mortality rate. Older people above 60 years with poor health conditions are more prone to mild infection and recovers within two weeks if treated timely [66].

SARS-CoV-2 virus (COVID-19) was originated from unknown sources that were expected as kinds of seafood. Despite passing several months in 2019, biomedical scientists or virologists are still under darkness about its mode of action. Naturally, there is enough panic due to unclear ways of virus attacks and subsequently, no such specific medicine or vaccine to cope with the situation.

How it Spread?

When a healthy person comes in close contact with a sick person, then through droplet infection, it transmits either through eyes, nose, and mouth or hands, contaminated objects, surfaces, or personal use items like utensils, tissues, lift buttons, electronic devices, cups, and pens [67].

There is no evidence found that it spreads through food. The other highly infectious viruses like SARS and MERS suggests that food is not the route of infection.

What are the symptoms associated with Corona Virus?

The common symptoms are like Flu or Cold, and it may become mild to severe

- Fever
- Cough
- Shortness of Breathe

80% mild to moderate cases like cough, fever, runny nose, headache, muscle pain, diarrhea, etc., can be managed through the home, 14% severe disease needs admission in the hospital and only 6% ICU. Admission.

The virus is highly contagious and can be tested by only a few specialized labs having Biosafety level 4 (BSL4) is handling the suspected cases only, so there is no requirement if you are suffering from fever or cough only if your doctor is recommended the testing should be done.

How long does it survive?

It survives up to 8-10 hours over porous surfaces like paper, wood, cardboard, sponge, and fabric and a little longer in nonporous surfaces like glass, plastics, metals, and varnished wood, and the only way to get rid of it is to disinfect the surface.

What Specimen is needed for Coronavirus?

CDC recommends Upper respiratory tract specimens (Nasopharyngeal and Oropharyngeal swabs) for preliminary testing. Patients with ventilator also lower respiratory tract specimens.

Prevalence:

Death rate with different viruses-

Novel   Corona Virus-2 %

Flu in USA-0.1%

Swine Flu-0.02%

SARS-9.6%

MERS-34%

Mortality Rate by Sex:

Male-4.7%

Female-2.8%

Mortality Rate by Age:

1. >80 Years-14.8%
2. 70-79 Years-8%
3. 60-69 Years-3.6%
4. 50-59 Years-1.3%
5. 40-49 Years-0.4%
6. 10-39 Years-0.2%
7. <10 Years-No Death

(Source: WHO & CDC).

Worldwide SARS-CoV involved 32 countries with 8422 confirmed cases and 916 causalities from Nov 2002 to Aug-2003.

MERS-CoV spread over 27 States involved. Two thousand four hundred ninety-six cases & 868 fatalities from April 2012 to Dec-2019. Novel CoronaVirus 2019 extends over 27 Countries with 34799 infected people and 724 in causalities from 29th Dec to Feb 2020 [67].

13. Some data analysis on COVID-19 prevalence (Cases) observed worldwide in graphical forms

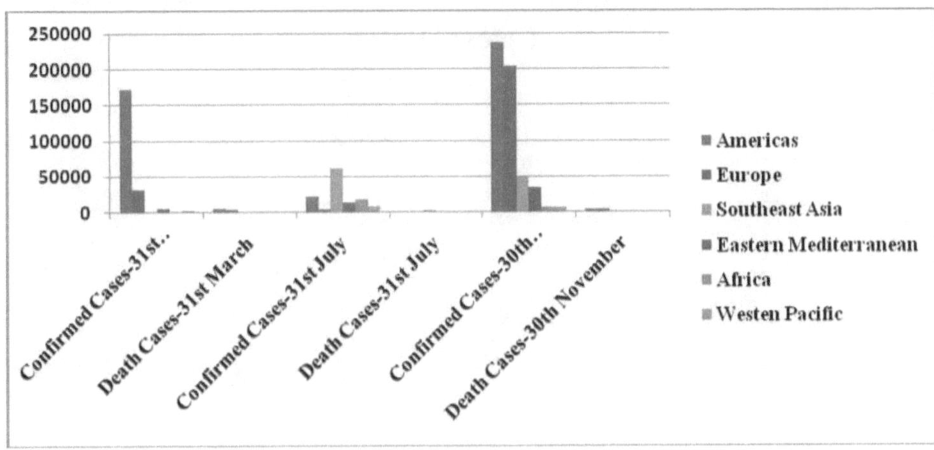

Fig.1: Confirmed Cases Vs. Death Cases due to COVID-19 zone wise, globally (March-November-20)

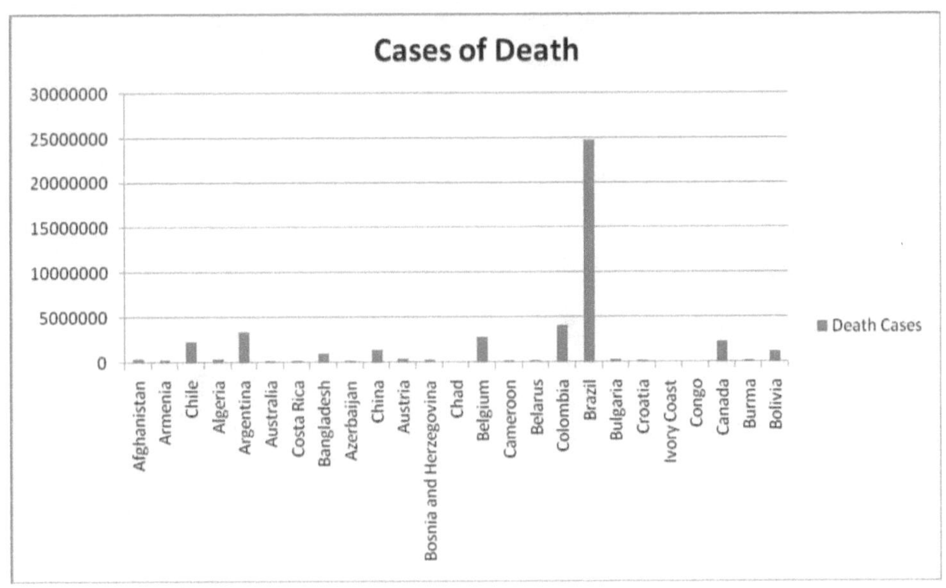

Fig.2: Country-wise Death Cases observed due to COVID-19

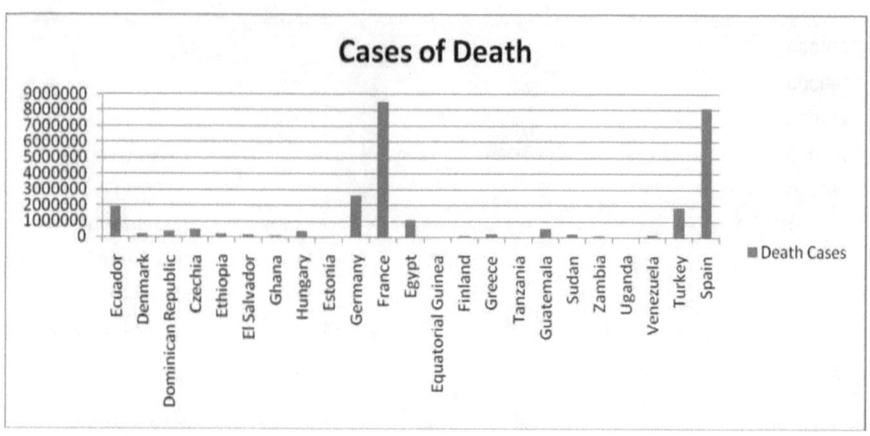

Fig.3: Country-wise Death Cases observed due to COVID-19

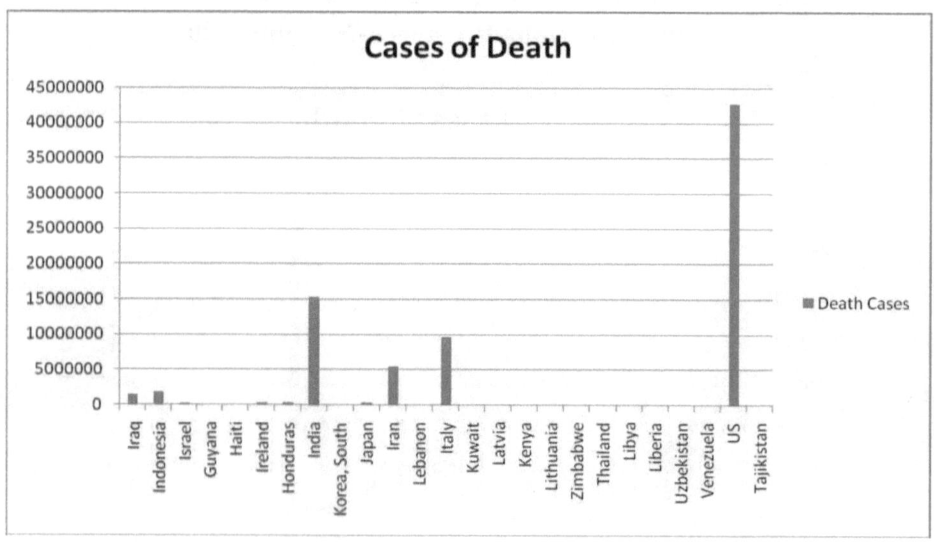

Fig.4: Country-wise Death Cases observed due to COVID-19

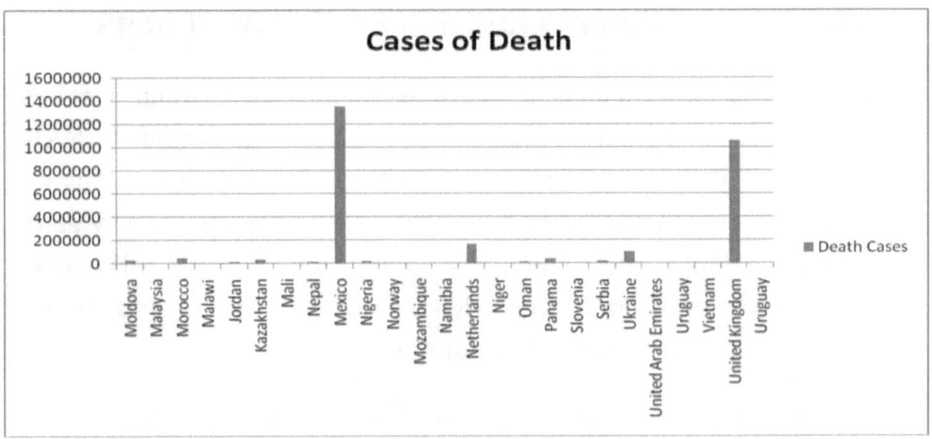

Fig.5: Country-wise Death Cases observed due to COVID-19

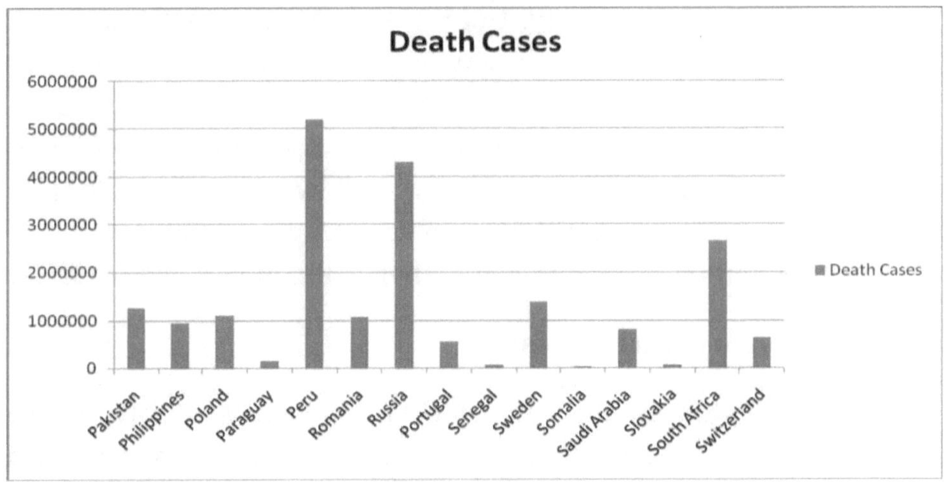

Fig.5: Country-wise Death Cases observed due to COVID-19

Disclaimer: All content related to diseases written here is based on general conditions but not for severity or any severe cases, .i.e. person to person variable. The Author is not responsible for any circumstances.

Note:

*

14. Possible Dietary Guidelines to follow at home

Here are a few dietary instructions to prevent Corona Virus by boosting your immune system as the infection is similar to SARS & MERS. On that evidence, the diet will be the same foods that enhance your immunity; boosting immunity is not a one day game; it takes a long time to improve your immunity. By following a healthy lifestyle and diet, sleep, reduced stress, and regular exercise, we can improve our immunity.

This infectious disease is new to all of us. We only improve our immune system by including eight micronutrients such as Vitamin A, C, D, E, folic acid, iron, zinc, and selenium, which play a vital role in boosting immunity. But there is no significant fact, and it works before catching and may help improve your condition by enhancing your immune power. We should supply all the eight nutrients regularly through our food by including five magic foods such as one amla/lemon per day, yellow and orange fruit or vegetables, Leafy green leafy vegetables, two portions of pulses, and one portion of sprouts, and lastly handful of nuts and seeds [69].

1) **Vitamin C Rich Foods:**

Vit C helps prevent the common cold, and there is no harm to take Vit-C up to 2000mg/d. It acts as an antioxidant as well as a cofactor of biosynthetic and gene regulatory enzymes. Foods rich in Vit-C are amla, lemon, citrus fruits, Guava, Tomato, Stawberries& Pineapple. We should consume it fresh in raw form as Vit-C is a heat liable vitamin.

2) **Vitamin A Rich Foods:**

Vit A is also A powerful antioxidant and anti-inflammatory vitamin, which is needed to maintain your immunity. We can include beta carotene-rich foods, which gets converted into Vit

A. The sound sources are yellow and orange fruits and vegetables like Carrot, Ripe Mango, Ripe Papaya, Ripe Tomato, Orange and Sweet potato, etc.

3) **Folic acid and Iron:** Green leafy vegetables like Agathi, Amaranthus, Colocasia leaves, Curry leaves, Drumstick leaves, Coriander leaves, Fenugreek leaves, Lettuce, Spinach, Mint, etc. are fair sources of folic acid and iron

4) **Vitamin E Rich Foods-** Nuts and seeds like Almonds, Peanut, Pistachio, pumpkin seeds, sunflower seeds, etc. are good sources of Vitamin E

5) **Vitamin-D Rich Foods:**
It is suitable for your health, protecting against respiratory tract infection. At least 15 mins of sun exposure daily, i.e., 2000 I.U./Day, is useful as many of us are Vit D deficient.

6) **Zinc**:
Zinc helps us protect from white blood cell infection and whoever is deficient in zinc is more susceptible to cold, flu, and other viruses like Covid-19. So, 40 mg of zinc may recommend avoiding flu-like infections. Good zinc sources are-Bengal gram, Black gram, Green gram, lentils, Red gram, and soybeans.

7) **Magnesium:**
Consuming adequate magnesium enhances a festive mood. Good magnesium sources are Whole grains such as oats, wheat bran, broccoli, raspberries, nuts & seeds, beans, bananas, and dark chocolate.

8) **Omega 3's**
Omega 3, like DHA, EPA & ALA, helps reduce body inflammation and improve your mood. Good sources are cold-water fish such as tuna, salmon, mackerel and some vegan microalgae, hemp seeds, chia seeds, pumpkin seeds, and dark green leafy vegetables like kale and spinach.

9) **Antioxidants and polyphenols:**

Antioxidants and polyphenols are the powerhouses that help in reducing inflammation and also improves gut flora. If possible, include either yellow or orange colored fresh fruits and vegetables like Carrot, Ripe Mango, Ripe Papaya, Ripe Tomato, Orange, and Sweet potato. Else include Vit E and selenium-rich nuts and seeds like walnut, almond, extra virgin olive oil, etc.

WHO suggests that instead of using supplements as an immunity booster, healthy food is better. Healthy foods improve our gut health due to a variety of microbiomes work as healthy microbiomes. Each type plays a different role in enhancing immunity and health as gut bacteria by producing some beneficial chemicals. They help in Vit A activation of food to maintain the immune system [69,70].

What to eat to feed your microbiome?

The best sources are a variety of plant-based foods, which are high in fiber and less processed. So, include plenty of fruits and vegetables and nuts and seeds: whole grains and healthy fats like olive oil. Try to limit extra salt, sweets, and sugary drinks, and also foods containing additives. You can include natural yogurt, curd, and fermented foods like kefir, pickles, kimchi, and sauerkraut, which act as probiotics and improve the microbiome [71].

Low Carbohydrate Diet:

There is no substantial evidence regarding a low carbohydrate diet. It helps in a healthy lifestyle and long term health benefits. But it appears that diabetics and persons with other metabolic disorders are at higher risk of Covid-19.

There is evidence that sugar impairs white blood cell function. We don't have any proof that reducing sugar can enhance your immune system, but it helps maintain blood sugar and decrease infection risk. One recent study showed that a keto diet helps infected mice with influenza to do the same for humans in Covid-19 [71,72].

15. Probable best foods to be included in the daily diets to combat

✓ **Turmeric:**

It contains the compound curcumin, which boosts the immune system, but there is no direct connection to viral infections.

✓ **Echinacea:**
An herb is showing evidence that it helps to fight the common cold. It can be safe to take for a short time for protection against Covid-19.

✓ **Garlic:**
It possesses an antibacterial and antiviral effect to fight against the common cold. But it needs so many trials to confirm whether it has any beneficial effects against respiratory tract infections, but it helps boost your immunity.

✓ **Broth and Chicken Soup:**
Broth and chicken soup prevents dehydration as well as soothes a sore throat, and relieves congestion. Few studies showed that taking chicken soup inhibits neutrophils' migration, indirectly improving our ability to heal the infection.

✓ **Yogurt:**
Fresh yogurt without added sugar helps in sore throat and also enhances your immune system.

✓ **Leafy Greens:**

Spinach, kale, and other leafy greens enhance your immune system when you have flu as they are rich in immune-enhancing nutrition like Vit C &Vit E.

✓ **Broccoli:**

It's rich in immune-boosting Vit C &Vit E along with calcium and fiber and can benefit your body when you have flu.

✓ **Oats:** A nutritious hot bowl of oatmeal is a natural source of immune boosters like Vit E, Polyphenol antioxidants, and Beta-glucan fiber.

✓ **Spices:**

Few spices such as pepper, horseradish, cardamom avoid congestion and improve breathing.

✓ **Proper Hydration:**

Be hydrated and include ginger tea, herbal tea, lemon tea, honey, coconut water, lemon juice, etc.

Besides, this avoids a thing that lowers your immune system:

✓ Alcohol
✓ Caffeinated beverages
✓ Crunchy crackers, chips
✓ Processed foods

Other Recommendations:

There is no specific magic food that protects you from Coronavirus, so only healthy eating may improve the condition and prevent and boost your immune system. Include plenty of fruits, vegetables, and seeds, but there is no direct connection to whether it truly helps or not. But regular consumption of fruits and vegetables shows a better immune response to pneumonia patients and reduces viral infection chances. We cannot conclude any specific fruits, but rainbow fruits provide adequate micronutrients, and these are also natural food and improve your overall health.

Whether fasting helps in Recovery?

One study showed intermittent fasting restores immune function. But during an acute pandemic, fasting is not a good idea as there is a higher risk of infection when you are hungry.

Take-home messages:

- ✓ Eating a healthy, nutritious diet minimizes your sugar level.
- ✓ Enough sleep for rejuvenation
- ✓ Manage your stress level
- ✓ Quit Smoking
- ✓ Regular Exercise
- ✓ Have sunshine and fresh air

Is meat Safe?

It is suspected that the animal may originate from Covid-19. But it is not transmitted through eating meat. WHO recommended cooking meat in high flame for 30 minutes and avoided eating raw and meat from diseased to kill all viruses. Everyone should maintain good personal hygiene when handling and preparing meat. Fearing the false outbreak, people avoid consuming meat and poultry. People even preferring a vegetarian diet. But the question is whether doing this protects you against this infectious Coronavirus disease.

Coronavirus is an upper respiratory tract infection and transmits through droplets. There is no relation that any virus or novel coronavirus is present in chicken, meat, or seafood and makes it unsuitable for consumption. There is no harm to take thoroughly washed and properly cooked meat as it effectively kills the SARS Virus, which is almost similar to Covid-19.

Avoid Consuming raw and unpasteurized milk and undercooked meat.

Myths Or Facts:

- ✓ Oregano oil proves effective against Coronavirus
- ✓ Taking Vit C and avoiding spicy food may help
- ✓ Avoiding cold drinks, milkshakes, or ice cream, there is nothing relating to this current virus.

16. WHO recommended nutritional guidelines for adults during the Covid-19 outbreak [73,74]

Proper nutrition with a well-balanced diet along with food is essential to stay away from infectious disease.

- ✓ Eat fresh and unprocessed foods every day
- ✓ Include plenty of fruits and vegetables, legumes, nuts, whole grains, oats, brown rice, roots and tubers, egg, and milk-
    - At least five servings of vegetables
    - 180 Gm of grains
    - 160 Gm of Non-Veg twice a week
    - Egg white twice or thrice a week
- ✓ Do not overcook the vegetables as overcooking losses vitamins
- ✓ If choosing dried fruits and vegetables, opt without added salt and sugar
- ✓ Drink sufficient water
- ✓ Avoid caffeine, sweetened juices, and sugary drinks
- ✓ Include unsaturated fats (olive, soy, canola, nuts, corn oil, sunflower oils instead of saturated fats like butter, ghee, dalda, cheese, palm oil, etc.
- ✓ Include Low-fat dairy

- ✓ Avoid Trans fats found in processed foods like pizza, cookies, fried foods, etc.
- ✓ Eat less sugar and salt

What About Fasting?

One study showed intermittent fasting restores immune function. But during an acute pandemic, fasting is not a good idea as there is a higher risk of infection when you are hungry.

Overall dietary guidelines:

- ✓ Eating a healthy, nutritious diet minimizes your sugar level and indirectly prevents Coronavirus as diabetics are more prone to Coronavirus.
- ✓ Enough sleep for rejuvenation
- ✓ Manage your stress level
- ✓ Quit smoking
- ✓ Regular exercise
- ✓ Have sunshine and fresh air
- ✓ Avoid foods that lower your immune system like- alcohol, caffeinated beverages, crunchy crackers, chips, processed foods.

There is no specific magic food that protects you from Coronavirus, so only healthy eating may improve the condition and prevent and boost your immune system.

WHO Recommended [74]

- ✓ Washing hands before touching raw and cooked foods
- ✓ Covering your mouth and nose while sneezing and coughing
- ✓ Keeping distance with everyone having respiratory problems like coughing and sneezing

✓ All utensils which are to be used for eating and drinking should be clean and sanitized before use. Cleaning should be done in hot water for 35 minutes in 75 degrees Celcius

Myths and Facts:

- Oregano oil proves effective against Coronavirus
- Taking Vitamin C and avoiding spicy food control virus
- Avoiding cold drinks, milkshakes, or ice cream, but the fact is there is no relation between all these myths about Coronavirus.

17. Few nutritional Tips that will be beneficial to prevent Coronavirus [75,76]

As these are effective against other flu-like SARS and MERS, it may be possible that these will be effective for the corona Virus.

✓ **Hydration**: Our body is composed of almost 75 percent of water, and a regular intake of 8 glasses is recommended, but as during these days we are less physically active and not feeling thirsty, so it is essential to take care of your body by hydrating yourself even if you are not feeling thirsty. If you don't like plain water, you can add flavors like lemon, orange, or cucumber but avoid sugary drinks. You can also include herbal tea, ginger tea, tulsi decoction, or even your homemade tea by adding cardamom, cinnamon, ginger, raw turmeric, mint or tulsi leaves, and anise.

✓ **Go Foods**: Foods that are rich in complex carbohydrates foods and are energy-dense foods like whole grain rice (brown rice), wholegrain pasta, bread, potato, corn, oatmeals, noodles, honey, and these foods keeps you full for longer times, i.e., it gives you a satiety feeling.

- ✓ **Grow Foods**: These foods help in faster Recovery and these are bodybuilding foods which repairs wear and tear of tissues and are mainly protein-rich foods like which needed in moderate amount, but it is necessary to include every day like Eggs, Milk, and products, fishes, beans, lentils, gelatine, soya beans, yogurt. The incredible amount of vitamins and minerals and the longer shelf-life of plant proteins show better immunity protection.
- ✓ **Glow Foods**: Colourful fruits and vegetables rich in vitamins cum other antioxidants help boost immunity capacity assuring ready to fight against any infection.
- ✓ **Green fruits and vegetables:** peas, cabbage, lettuce, broccoli, spinach, some sprouts, all types of beans, cucumbers, kiwi, lime, green/bell peppers, apples, green grapes, and avocados.
- ✓ **Fruits and vegetables (yellow and orange-colored):** pumpkin, corn (sweet), sweet potatoes, yellow pepper, tomatoes (yellow/red), carrots, oranges, apricots, grape, mangoes, peaches, ripe papayas, pineapple, and pears.
- ✓ **Red Fruits and vegetables:** radishes, red tomatoes, cabbage (red), beets roots, grapes, strawberries, watermelon, strawberries, raspberries, cherries, apples, and pomegranate
- ✓ **Blue and Purple fruits and vegetables:** Eggplant, purple-colored cabbage and potato, blueberries, plums, grapes (purples), blackberries, raisins, and other dry fruits and also figs.
- ✓ **Preserved fruits and vegetables:** pickled foods, dried, canned, fermented foods, and fair alternative sources of fresh fruits and vegetables as tasty ready preparations. These may bring not only taste and flavor but also antioxidants benefits
- ✓ **Fortified Foods:** Fortified foods help supply all nutrients when you cannot include varieties in your diet due to food insecurity.

✓ **Exercise:** WHO recommends a minimum of 30 minutes of exercise for every adult and 1 hour for every child. Either you can opt for yoga, dance, and use stairs instead of elevators.

✓ **Foods to avoid:**
  - High fat, sugar, and salt-rich
  - Processed foods
  - Foods with low or no nutrition like cake, candies, chips, sodas, potato chips, salted snacks, sweet desserts, fried and fast foods.

Does Corona Virus spread if an infected person handles or cooks the food? [76]

The answer is yes; it may transmit through droplets during coughing or sneezing. So, it is a good idea to avoid it.

General Food precautions:

- Frequent washing of hands with soap and water
- Soak all fruits and vegetables in lukewarm water for at least 30 minutes before cooking
- Avoid cooking if you are sick
- Avoid food from outside
- Avoid raw foods and foods from vendors

18. Can pregnant women pass Coronavirus to the unborn child?

There is no proper evidence of whether the virus is transmitted from a mother to an unborn child. Still, she should take appropriate precautions and visit medical care if suffering from fever, cough, breathing difficulty, etc.

Is it safe for a mother to breastfeed if she is infected with Coronavirus? [77-79]

All mothers whoever is having symptoms of cough, fever, and respiratory distress and are at risk and should start medical care as soon as possible. A mother can breastfeed their baby while following all required precautions like wearing masks when they are in close contact with their child, washing hands before starting feeding, and if a mother is too ill, she should feed her child by using a spoon. According to WHO, everyone should follow these preventive measures:

1) Avoid air travel
2) Avoid public gatherings
3) Hand washing using 20 seconds process
4) Use of hand sanitizers
5) Maintain 1 to 3 ft distance from persons suffering from cold and fever

19. Food industries - profit or loss during the pandemic [80-82].

- One of the hospitals uses a high dose of vitamin C as a treatment against Coronavirus, and a report from China that quantities are more than reference dietary intake.
- Nestle and Unilever are trying hard to support their suppliers and community globally
- Coronavirus will increase the sales of probiotic products due to increased demand for healthy foods
- Dairy products like Danone are helping to get out of the crisis, and their sales increased during the current crisis
- Butcher shops are looking for nonessentials
- The cold drinks and ice cream business is going down
- Sanitizer companies are gaining profit day by day
- Staple food price is hiking day by day
- Kellogg's companies are benefiting these days

- Confectionaries industries are suffering

20. Reasons not to use nasogastric tubes for Coronavirus

1. It is challenging to monitor tube placement in isolation
2. Patients who are already suffering from the sore throat are complaining of pain and may remove themselves, which becomes a cause of infection

Food that is considered acceptable during tube feeding:

- ✓ Milk-based fortified liquid diets which are easy to digest if not having lactose intolerance
- ✓ Potassium-rich unsweetened fruit juices
- ✓ Rice, Dalia, and oats gruel
- ✓ Vegetable soups

Disclaimer: All content related to diseases written here is based on general conditions but not for severity or any severe cases, .i.e. person to person variable. The Author is not responsible for any circumstances.

Part-III:

A few sample balanced diet plans for the patients suffering from lifestyle disorders as discussed in this book. The diet plans have been designed mainly for the people of India .

Disclaimer: All content related to diseases written here is based on general conditions but not for severity or any severe cases, .i.e. person to person variable. The Author is not responsible for any circumstances

Note:

i) A SAMPLE BALANCED DIET FOR THE PATIENT OF CORONARY HEART DISEASE

Age – 49 years, Height – 6ft=183 cm, weight – 104 kg, BMI – 31.04; **Diagnosis** (based on tests) – obesity stage-1, HTN, Hypertriglyceridemia/ Hyperlipidemia, slightly elevated TSH (subclinical hypothyroidism?), little, Low Vitamin D, mild, Fatty Liver. Target weight - 75(+/-)

So **104-75= 29 kg to lose**. @ 5kg x2 months = 10 kg; rest module, 3kg X6 months and entire period should be under dietitian's follow up. (Ref:18.5- 22.9=normal range); >22.9-24.9 <= overweight ; >25-29.9< = pre obesity ; >30-39.9< =obesity stage-I ; >40-49.9< = Obesity Stage II,; and above 50< = morbid stage As per Asian Value.

Tests: High TGL, LDL, TSH, AST, ALT, low Vit-D

Diet Type - Low Salt, Low Carbs, Low Animal Protein & Very Low Fat Diet.

<u>Soft cum Bland Diet- No spices, significantly less oil, More soluble fibers.</u>

Tentative Exercise plan :

1 hour of daily **exercises is preferable in the early morning to come down weight by safe method & retain for future.**

(**avoidance** > subject to any injury/ surgery/pregnancy/ knee or joint pain/arthritis/osteoarthritis). Presently to practice at home or home campus only. Supplements all commercial are not safe rather harmful severely, But if no such work out, no results or delayed results.)

<u>Tentative Diet Plan (30days-weekly plan)</u>

(Reference 2300 kcal/day for sedentary man as per ICMR-NIN)

**make a daily plan as per your family routine.
All raw weight calculation, before cooking,**

Monitor weight every @ 7day till one month./next review.

Daily Calorie Requirement – 1600kcal/day by foods & 1 hour of early morning daily exercises to come down weight by safe method & retain for future. Supplements all commercial are not safe rather harmful severely.

Calorie Segregation :

1.Carbohydrate – 1600kcal x 55% = 880 kcal/4 = 220gm

2.Protien- 1600kcal x 20%) = 320kcal/4 = 80gm

3.Fat -15% -   1600kcal X 15% = 240kcal /9 = 26ml.< (only cooking oil 2-3tsf)

4. Fiber through fresh fruits and vegetables 1600X10% = 160 Kcal/day

<u>No Butter, Ghee, all high fats, etc. as these all are highly restricted for you) Preferably Olive oil Or sun drop heart</u>

<u>TENTATIVE DIET PLAN</u> (for 30days)

Rotational and calculations based on raw ingredients

Advice: Low fat, low carbs, high fiber, timely low calorie eating with dynamic lifestyles

Wake up: 5.30/6 am – After refreshments, 20gm CHIA seeds (raw and black available in spencer/Online, make ready dust for 1 week) + 5gm methi dust add in 1 glass lukewarm water (300 ml) +

20 ml=2 tbsp Alevera Juice (Appoloo/Dabur).- drink entire sharbat as detox water.

After 5 Min = Have 5 gm raw Garlic at almost empty stomach

After 30min- enough water + 1 Cream cracker Biscuit + 1 cup green tea-

7 am- Indoor exercises –practice for 15 min as per the time available & also at evening. Practise exercises at bed or floor – Yogas/prayamanas.

7.30 am-Outdoor Exercises (safe distancing/as possible) - 30 min walking but not running /or heavy strenuous + free hand at home campus 15min. total = 15+30+15=60 min. or minimum 45 min for total 3 types exercises.

8 am You can also have enough water + 5 gm raw garlic it is not already taken.

8.30 am- (not mandatory but may have on Holidays) 2 cream cracker Marie Britannia + some water + 1 cup green tea.

Breakfast– (alternate day) at home/ out – Not chilled foods

1) Plain oats meal 50 gm +100 gm mix green vegetables/raw curd 30gm.
2) 2 pcs roasted brown bread + plain curd 30gm/Veg. Sandwich 1 pc (if out)
3) Poha/Upma 50gm + 50gm green salad.+ 30 gm curd (out)
4) Sattu 30 gm sarbat added with pink salt+ some black pepper (out) + 1 egg white (3-4/pc **egg white** per week may be added during snacks)

10 am – **(not mandatory** /at the office) some water + 1 cup green tea with one Biscuit available in the office.

11.30 am – 100 gmx2= 200gm total= 1 guava/ 5pcs berries / 1 apple (NO Banana /dry fruits/ sweet all juices) + 1 any citrus fruit like 100 gm mosambi /pineapple.

1.30 pm –Lunch (all soft boil, very low salt, sugar, and spices) – 500Kcal. (5days/week) – 30 gm soft white rice (basmati 4-5days/week) or 1 small cup=50 gm brown rice (2 days /week) / if out better **2 pcs polka roti** + 20 gm mug dal +100 gm vegetables + one pc. egg white. (3 days/week); chicken-2day 100gm leg pc strew type., Avoid red meat like Goat/Turkey etc/much animal/organic food).

veg thali - >50gm (**2days/week**) = 2 cube plain paneer (without cream) can add green salad 50gm or more + sour curd /raita 50gm/ also can add 20gm Tarka/rajma/posto/soya 5pc.). Same vegetables strew not curry/gravy must there in Dinner also.

Drink water after 20 min of Lunch and eat <u>foods by proper chewing</u>.

4 pm (not mandatory) -any- 2pcs citrus fruit like grapes, orange/ Berries/Avocado/Guava, etc. (Total 300gm fruits per day better).

No fruits in the evening. Take before 4 pm. Or 11 am or 4 pm, Not early morning or evening or night time.

5 pm – 6 pm or 6 pm-7 pm – some mild walking and freehand exercise inside the home campus.

5.30/6 pm – at OFFICE (Not mandatory)- 1 Cream cracker biscuit + 1 cup of green tea/black tea.

7/8 pm- evening – Any light calorie meal – 2 pcs Idly/ chira/muri 50gm with chana/salad, e.g., beet carrot, cucumber slices. Avoid all junk/fried foods/Green chilly 1pc but no other fried.

10 pm – Dinner: As Lunch, fresh cooking, lukewarm, not chilled/spicy. Avoid rice, Only 2phulka roti (2-3days/week) /Dalia 50 gm (4-5days/week) –RICE if not taken during lunch but prefer without rice here + 20gm dal + 100gm mix veg soft boiled (without potatoes, etc.) + *No Animal Foods at Night.*

VEG (5-7 days in a week) – Can add - paneer (no cream) 50gm= 2-3 small pcs (less calorie similar as lunch).

By 11 pm max sleep – No late or stress or mental pressure. Avoid late-night work. Drink water after 20 min and practice some yoga before bedtime.

Total Intake as Kcal: 1650 (+/-50Kcal) and work out expenditure = 600Kcal (+/-50kcal) if completed as per advice/day

Some primary Advice mainly to follow

- Buy a kitchen weight machine for precise weight of rice, wheat, dal, etc. all staple foods to restrict calories.,
- Add a little more garlic in Your chicken strew/ sabzi daily, but it must be fresh eating. Black pepper also helpful.
- Avoid alcohol and smoking and all fried or fast foods.
- Use sunflower cooking oil max 3- tbsp.= 30 ml per day Or use Olive oil
- Drink water a full 3 ltr and drink after 20-30min followed by your Lunch or dinner.
- Should NOT have chilled or too hot foods. No need for any health drinks or protein drink
- Seven aprx sleep per day. Sleep at night only, not day time.
- Exercises outdoor safely & Indoor as more possible 1 hr or 400 minutes min. in week hours in total by early morning

and evening both time. OR you can do it frequently in a whole day @ 15 min.

Best exercises during COVID crisis, gentle walking, freehand, some yogas, pranayamas, But Not Any Outside Gatherings. Check email attached files.

- Always movements oriented and plenty of water 3-4 ltr in the summertime.
- Sweet water fresh fishes you can have NON-veg days/week
- Avoid or very low Potatoes, Sweet potatoes or other, allergic vegetables if you have, have more green and fresh.
- During the 1st month, prefer roti or Dalia at night dinner, else you should eat brown rice available 30 gm average not more till advice, alter, any change other rice types.
- Better add roti max 3-4 pcs to avoid fat—fewer moistures. Avoid maida or other oily foods, including parantha, for acidity, GERD.
- Avoid all packed masalas and use only turmeric, garlic, phoron, black pepper, little onion, rock salt 5 gm, and cooking oil as reasonable.
- Avoid elachi, bay leaves, hing, sauces, kasandi, all packet spices. Etc.
- Presently avoid excess eggs, chicken, and no mutton even at home.

<u>Some Important Advice</u>

#Take maximum greens & green vegetables like gourd family (ash gourd, bitter gourd, ridge gourd, etc.) in addition to methi, parwal, soft beans (seem, data, etc.). All green salad like capsicum, cucumber, beet, carrot, allowed.

No potatoes & underground vegetables, pumpkin, Brinjal, Kachu, SAAG. Spinach, Broccoli, Raddish, Cauliflower, Cabbage, etc.

<u>Best vegetables to eat as mixed vegetables.</u>

Beetroots, Beet, Carrots, Capsicum, All gourd family vegetables like bitter gourd, ridge gourd, Bottle gourd,

<u>Best Fruits to eat</u>

All citrus fruits like Musambi, Lemon, Orange, 1+1pc, all berries, Pear, Apple, Guava are good fiber-rich.

NO banana, all dry fruits sweet, mangoes, grapes, dates, nuts, raisins, dry dates, coconut, etc., can not be consumed for 1-2 months.

Very Low or restrictions

Street foods, occasional fatty foods, Junk, creamy, spicy, oily foods & high-calorie all snacks.

- Avoid rajma, Tarka, soy, soy products, all dal pulses except Moong/Arajhar dal allowed. Eggs, Mutton, Red meats all.
- Avoid mustard oil or similar all seeds oil like soya, sunflower oil, Only use Rice bran oil or better can afford Olive Oil for PUFA-Good fat)
- NO Coffee, Brinjal, Coconut, spices, street foods. Junk, creamy foods.
- No cows/Buffaloes milk, no full cream or similar,
- Salt below 4gm, raw sugar, if non-diabetic 2 tbsp= max 30gm.

---

ii) A SAMPLE BALANCED DIET FOR THE PATIENT OF DYSLIPIDEMIA

Age – 27 years, Height – 169 cm, weight – 77 kg, BMI – 26.92 (27). **Diagnosis** (based on tests) – Pre-obesity, Hyperlipidemia, Hypertension, Target weight **- 63(+/-),** Target weight 63; So **80-63= 17 kg to lose**. @ 5kg x2 months = 10 kg;+ rest 4kg X2 months and entire period should be under dietitian's follow up. (Ref: 18.5-22.9=normal range); >22.9-24.9 <= overweight ; >**25-29.9**< = pre obesity ; >30-39.9< =obesity stage-I ; >40-49.9< = Obesity Stage II,; and above 50< = morbid stage As per Asian Value.

Tests: High TGL & LDL, high B.P

Diet Type - Low Salt, Low Carbs, Protein & Very Low Trans & Sat Fat Diet.

Tentative Exercise plan :

1 hour of daily **exercises to come down weight by safe method & retain for future. (avoidance >** subject to any injury/ surgery/pregnancy/ knee or joint pain/arthritis/osteoarthritis). Presently to practice at home or home campus only. Supplements all commercial are not safe rather harmful severely)

Soft cum Bland Diet- No spices, significantly less oil, low salt – More soluble fibers with low purine).

Tentative Diet Plan (30days-weekly plan)

(Reference 2300 kcal/day for sedentary man as per ICMR-NIN)

**make a daily plan as per your family routine.
All raw weight calculation, before cooking,**

Monitor weight every @ 7day till 1 month./next review.

Daily Calorie Requirement – 1600kcal/day by foods & 1 hour of early morning daily exercises to come down weight by safe method & retain for future.

Supplements all commercial are not safe rather harmful severely.

Calorie Segregation :

1.Carbohydrate – 1600kcal x 55% = 880 kcal/4 = 220gm

2.Protien- 1600kcal x 20%) = 320kcal/4 = 80gm

3.Fat -15% -   1600kcal X 15% = 240kcal /9 = 26ml.< (only cooking oil 2-3tsf)

4. Fiber by fresh fruits and vegetables 1600X10% = 160 Kcal/day

No Butter, Ghee, all high fats, etc., as these all are highly restricted for you.) Preferably Olive oil Or sun drop heart

<u>TENTATIVE DIET PLAN </u>(for 30days)

Rotational and calculations based on raw ingredients

Advice: Low fat, low carbs, high fiber, timely low calorie eating with dynamic lifestyles

Wake up: 6 am – 10gm CHIA seeds (raw and black available in spencer/Online) + 5gm methi add in 1 glass water (300 ml) + 2-3 drops Lemon apple cider vinegar.- drink entire sarbat as detox water.

After 30min- enough water + 1 cup green tea

6.30/7 am- Indoor exercises –practice for 30 min as per the time available & also in the evening. Practise exercises at bed or floor –

Yogas/prayamanas.

7.30 am-Outdoor Exercises (safe distancing) - 30 min walking/mild running + free hand at home campus 15min. total = 30+30+15=75min.

during running and freehand exercises, # must have a handful of water-soaked sprouts + 5 gm raw garlic.

8 am -Then take 10 min rest & enough water.

8.31am- 2 cream cracker Marie Britannia + some water + 1 cup green tea.

9.am – Breakfast– <u>(change every alternate day) at home/ out</u>

5) Plain oats meal 50 gm +100 gm mix vegetables/plain curd 30gm.
6) 2 pcs roasted brown bread + plain curd 30gm/Veg. Sandwich 1 pc (out)
7) Poha/Upma 50gm + green salad.+ 30 gm curd (out)
8) Sattu 30 gm sarbat added with pink salt+ some black pepper (out)

10 am – (not mandatory)some water + 1 cup green tea or half glass mosambi juice if possible.

11.30 am – 100 gm= 1 guava/ berries / 1 apple (NO Banana /dry fruits/ sweet all juices) + 1 any citrus fruit like 100 gm mosambi /pineapple

12/1 pm –Lunch – 30 gm soft white rice (basmati 4-5days/week) or 1 small cup=50 gm brown rice (2 days /week) / if out better **2-3pcs pholka roti** +

20 gm mug dal +100 gm mix veg. (less oil & spices –only

homemade) + 100 gm fresh fish- rohu/catla only fish but avoid curry/gravy etc. (5 days/week);

Avoid chicken, eggs, Avoid red meat/much animal/organic foods).

If veg thali - >50gm (**2days/week**) = 2 cube plain paneer (without cream) can add green salad + sour curd /raita 50gm/ also can add 20gm tarka/rajmah/posto/soya 5pc.).

Drink water after 20 min of lunch and eat foods by proper chewing.

4 pm – (**not mandatory**) -any- 2pcs citrus fruit like grapes, orange, small amla

No fruits in the evening. Take before 4 pm. Or 11 am or 4 pm, Not early morning or evening or night time.

5 pm – 6 pm or 6 pm-7 pm – some gentle walking and freehand exercise inside the home campus.-If Possible, Else At Morning Habits

5.30/6 pm – 1 Cream cracker biscuit + 1 cup of green tea/black tea.

7 pm- evening – Any light calorie meal – 2 pcs Idly/ chira/muri 50gm with chana/salad, e.g., beet carrot, cucumber slices.

9.30 pm – Dinner- Only 3phulka roti (2-3days/week) /Dalia 50 gm (4-5days/week) – No RICE + 20gm dal + 100gm mix veg soft boiled (without potatoes etc) + *No Animal Foods at Night.*

VEG (5-7 days in a week) – Can add - paneer (no cream) 50gm= 2-3 small pcs OR almost same low-calorie diet as like lunch.

If non-veg is not taken in lunch, then you can have 50 gm without curry fish.

By 11 pm max sleep – No late or stress or mental pressure

Some Important Advice

#Take maximum greens & green vegetables like gourd family (ash gourd, bitter gourd, ridge gourd, etc.) in addition to methi, parwal, soft beans (seem, data, etc.). All green salad like capsicum, cucumber, beet, carrot, allowed.

No potatoes & underground vegetables, pumpkin, Brinjal, Kachu, SAAG. Spinach, Broccoli, Raddish, Cauliflower, Cabbage, etc.

Best vegetables to eat as mixed vegetables.

Beetroots, Beet, Carrots, Capsicum, All gourd family vegetables like bitter gourd, ridge gourd, Bottle gourd,

Best Fruits to eat

All citrus fruits like Musambi, Lemon, Orange, 1+1pc, all berries, Pear, Apple, Guava are good fiber-rich. Avoid banana; all dry fruits sweet, mangoes, grapes, dates, nuts, raisins, dry dates, coconut, etc., can not be consumed for 1-2 months.

Note:

*

*

*

*

*

*

---

iii) A SAMPLE BALANCED DIET FOR THE PATIENT OF DIABETES MELLITUS

Age – 73, Male, Howrah, Height -161cm. Current weight–54 Kg.

BMI – 28 (Ref: 18.5-24.9); Foods habits –Non.veg

Working habits – Retired person, sedentary lifestyles

Diagnosis: Diabetes-II (HbA1C= 6.9%),
pre-obese stage -I, Acidity

Advice: Low Carbohydrate, DM Diet (for 30days)
Aprx. **calorie- 1400kcal/Day**

Classification of Nutrients based on total calorie:
(Raw/Uncooked ingredients)

1. Carbohydrate (CHO) – 1400 x 50% = 700Kcal /4 = 175gm
(-/+10gm)
3. Protein – (Mostly Plant based) – 1400 X 30% = 420/4 =
105gm (-/+5gm)
Fat (edible oil) 1400 X 15% = 210/9= 23ml/gm
(3TSF. (-/+2gm/ml)
4. Extra fiber-rich fruits and vegetables = 5%.

All uncooked raw calculation.

6 am -After rising – 300ml water +10 gm methi water(fenugreek) dust + 10gm chia seeds duly dust and soaked (Chia seeds available online/Spencer raw black costs approx 160/-, if you do not like chia seeds like in sharbat then may add in mix sabzi at lunch and dinner)

6.15 am-7 am maximum min and after dinner. #Avoid poses that are painful for chronic issues like spondylitis/if severe pain in the body but better results if you can practice as discussed for DM and Diabetic.

7 am- Then take 10 min rest & drink one glass water + 2 cream cracker Biscuit + 1 cup green or black tea.

7.15 am-7.45 am Outdoor Exercises -Then start walking 30 mins (1.5km to 2 km or max 30-45 min. walking on a day at home campus/non-crowded area).

8.30am– Breakfast – Rotational -1 menu 2days/week (/ means option as any')

1. 2 slice Brown breads + 1 glass skimmed/fat free milk 250 ml/Mix boil vegetables + 3 tbsp Curd (Doi)
2. 50gm Oatmeal with + 1 glass skimmed/fat free milk 250 ml/mix boil vegetables + 3 tbsp Curd (Doi)
3. 50 gm Poha or Porridge (no nuts/oil) + 100 gm mix boil vegetables + 3 tbsp Curd (Doi)
4. 1 veg. sand witch (50 gm raw) + 250ml milk/Mix veg, 50 gm curd

    # low oil 1 cup mix soft vegetables 50 -100 gm OR Curd 50gm raw curd/ raita OR 250 ml milk must be added with cereal based (left side) item. No chilled / cold foods from refrigerator.

9 am – some water &1 cup green /Liker tea/ lemon tea/black coffee at home. (not mandatory).

10/11 am –Snacks -1 guava/1 apple/5pcs. berries/,1 /pear + 1 Orange (as available)

12/1 pm –Lunch (4days/week) –preferably 50gm brown rice (Brown rice should in water-soaked for the last day-night for quickly boil and avoid white rice) + 100gm veg. serving or better take everyday bitter gourd recipe 100 gm +20 gm moong dal with soup + (sukta= papaya + badi+ bitter gourd, methi leaves/dust)

If Non-veg. (4days) + 1pc.50gm fish (Rohu/Catla) or 1-day chicken if you like (Boneless Chicken breast/leg pc 1/week.). Suggested to avoid white rice for one month

If veg. (3days/week) : 50gm plain paneer, just add some (100 gm) + raita: 50gm./salad (curd max 100 gm per day).

Do plan in a changing pattern/like school routine) .It depends upon Holiday but keeping in mind mostly working day. If the office in the home. Nearby then manage lunch at home.

Then –30 min. Gentle walking within home /campus followed by 10 min some sitting rest. No sleep or extended sitting after Lunch

3/4 pm – Green Tea or any fruit

5-6 pm- preferably mild walking30 min FRESH AIR AREAS.

7 pm –evening –green salad 50gm, etc. + sprouts (No salt). OR 2 idly with sambar no coconut chutney. After/during office or at home to eat these items,

7.30 pm: Then - can have 2 pcs cream cracker Biscuits + green/Liker tea/Ginger tea.

9 pm –Dinner – prefer 2 roti (4days/week) OR Dalia 50 gm (3days/week) ,(No rice) +15gm mug/arahar dal+ 50 gm mix veg (as Lunch) + salad 50gm

If interested 2 days non-veg then may have small pc fish -50 gm as lunch./1 Egg White.

VEG (mostly all days/5days/week): paneer 20gm=2 cubes or Tarka/sprouts 30 gm apart from above dal and sabzi.

10 pm –Some mild walking/ yogas,. Avoid stress and no overnight/ late night work.

<u>Very Low or restrictions</u>

Street foods, occasional fatty foods, Junk, creamy, spicy, oily foods & high-calorie all snacks.

- Avoid rajma, Tarka, soy, soy products, all dal pulses except Moong/Arajhar dal allowed. Eggs, Mutton, Red meats all.
- Avoid mustard oil or similar all seeds oil like soya, sunflower oil, Only use Rice bran oil or better can afford Olive Oil for PUFA-Good fat)
- NO Coffee, Brinjal, Coconut, spices, street foods. Junk, creamy foods.
- No cows/Buffaloes milk, no full cream or similar,
- Salt below 4gm, raw sugar, if non-diabetic 2 tbsp= max 30gm.
- Avoid all fried sweets or high-calorie sugar-rich sweets.
- Avoid Hilsha, prawn, egg yolk, rai, Millet, raw wheat (only refined/multi-grain atta). No maida. Lucchi, Parantha. In case you get all these.
- Avoid excess seeds, beans, or old backdated vegetables,
- Avoid all red seeds or blacks seeds or rotten or frozen foods; always consume fresh current- dated foods.

***Disclaimer**: All content related to diseases written here is based on general conditions but not for severity or any severe cases, .i.e. person to person variable. The Author is not responsible for any circumstances.*

Note:

iv) A SAMPLE BALANCED DIET FOR THE PATIENT OF HYPERTENSION

Male – 53 Yr., Height – 5'5" (165cm), Weight – 55 Kg. BMI - 20.22

Diagnosis – Hypertension, Hyperuricemia, high creatinine, Type – Diabetes. Current Tests Reports : (As per data available).

Serum Urea – 108 (Ref : 14-40mg/dl), Serum Creatinine – 5.1 (Ref : 0.7 – 1.4 mg/dl).Serum U.A – 6.8, Potassium - 5.0 –Higher side, CL- 107.6 – more

Recommended Diet Type: DASH diet, Low protein (40gm) for 1month, Low Sodium, Type II Diabetic Diet Plan with water limitation (some modifications done as per the last prescription).

Net Energy – 1400Kcal/Day , Carbohydrate –65% = 230gm , Protein 10% =35gm(mostly veg. sources recommended),Visible Fat – 38gm. (All inclusive supplement).   PENTASURE –DM is highly recommended @ 30gm = 2tbsp/ per serving twice on a day (initially can start @ 40gm/day ,then up to 60gm total /day).

TENTATIVE DIET PLAN   (30 days under observation)

(On Weekly Basis, you can organize/shuffle day today as per your convenience but not change the quantity, ingredients/meals, etc

6.30 am - Methi tasted the water (water 100ml only = small half tea cup+ 10gm methi dust filter, do not eat solid methi).

6.45 am – some steps mild walking to control sugar (Not heavy/ NOT speed exercises).

7.00 am – 1 cream cracker (Britannia) with small cup Liker tea.

8/9 am – Breakfast

Options: 1) 30gm plain Oatmeal with small Katori mix whole skin vegetables. OR

2) 1-2 Pcs Phulka Roti with mix green vegetables.

3) Low salt Muri / roasted chira (rice flakes) with 2-3 pcs cucumber/ fruit salad (as listed)

4) 20gm sattu sharbat, Or small quantity rice with vegetables./ small 30gm Dalia.

10.30 am – Pentasure- DM 20-30gm with little water.

11 am – 2 pcs fruits: 1 small normal level Guava, 2-3 papaya, 1 small apple berries. (NOT ALL citrus fruits, banana, high-calorie fruits including dry fruits, nuts all**)**

12/1 Pm – Lunch: 30gm basmati rice + 1-2 pcs Phula Roti, + 15 gm Mung dal soupy,+ 1-2 Katori soft gourds mix vegetables (homemade curry), + green salad small cup, + 50gm fresh fish Gada pc only new quality (avoid all seafood salted, flat. fishes). Avoid eggs, chicken.

3-4 pm - 2 cream cracker Biscuits or 1-2 pcs fruits as listed.
50C

6/7 pm – some evening good quality snacks (like Breakfast).

Like: Low salt Muri. Clean roasted chira with small quantity salad Or 30gm plain Oat with boil dry vegetables. (No fast foods/ fried foods).

8 Pm - Pentasure- DM 20-30gm with little water.

9.Pm – Dinner :

2-3 Pcs Roti + 15 gm Mug dal, 1-2 Katori green mix vegetables prefer- gourds veg. with Karela separately., cucumber 2 slices, sometimes 50gm fresh rohu fish (no chicken/ meat/ animal others foods).

10 Pm – Tight sleep & wake up again next day on time.

Avoid Strictly :

High Urea Foods

- Not: XX meat, fish, chicken, eggs, cheese, milk, and yogurt
- Salt and Salty Foods, Chips, etc.
- Processed meats such as deli meats, bacon, sausage, and ham. Canned soups, frozen dinners, pickles, and olives are also high in sodium and should be avoided.
- Large Portions of Protein include meat, poultry, seafood, beans, milk, grains and vegetables, poultry, milk, or soy foods.
- Avoid – soy foods, soybeans, all beans, broccoli, local greens (sag), spinach, reddish, pumpkin, all old seeds black seeds or red seeds including tomatoes similar vegetables, etc., avoid Potatoes, Sweet Potatoes, all roots, stream (Kachu types) .brinjal,
- It's better to cook with bottle gourd, Karela, papaya, capsicum, all greens soft skin vegetables as per listed can add some beet, carrots.
- Avoid Onion, high garlic, all spices which are rich in dried powder types. Avoid all packed masalas.

Foods High in Potassium

NOT X high in potassium such as avocados, bananas, oranges,

prunes, potatoes, spinach, tomatoes, beans, and brown rice.

Foods High in Phosphorus

NOT X avoid including whole-grain bread, bran cereal, high oatmeal, nuts, sunflower seeds, and colas.

DIET SHOULD BE: HELPFUL

1. Arrange a low-protein diet.

2. For weakness & supplement, add Pentasure –DM (for diabetic)

3. Develop a low-sodium diet – low table salt below 2 gm <

4. Helpful: cranberry, pomegranate, cucumber, bitter gourd, etc., can help stimulate the kidneys to excrete more urea. So, patients with high urea levels can eat more of these foods, but they should pay attention to their potassium level.

5.**Watch & Limit your fluid intake.** As a general rule, you can drink six to eight water glasses each day or doctor's advice.

6. **Restrict your activity level.** Exercise can still offer essential health benefits overall, so you may not want to exclude it from your routine completely. You should NOT practice high-intensity exercises. Instead of running, try mild level 10-15 min walking or practicing yoga.

7. **Sleep well.** -7 - 8 hours deep sleep. Not late night work/ stress.

8. **Increase your consumption of plant-based foods.** Vegetarian diets are often recommended to bring down high creatinine levels and reduce kidney disease risk due to high blood pressure or diabetes.

__Disclaime__r: All content related to diseases written here is based on general conditions but not for severity or any severe cases, .i.e. person to person variable. The Author is not responsible for any circumstances.

Note :

v) A SAMPLE BALANCED DIET FOR THE PATIENT OF GALL BLADDER DISEASE

Age – 26years, male, Height – 5.7 Ft =171 cm; Present Weight – 43 kg. BMI – 14.88 (Range – 18.5-24.9), Foods Habits – all types

Diagnosis -. Severe undernutrition. 14.88 severe≤16-Moderate -16.9 <17 mild undernutrition <18.5 – 24.9 normal range >overweight.

Diet -   High Protein Very Low Fat Diet
Recommended Energy – 2400kcal/day.
(for 30-45 days, after may be modified)

1. Carbohydrate –   2400 X 60% =   1440 / 4 = 360gm./day
Mostly in staple meals (cereals -rice, refined wheat-avoid gluten)
2. Protein - 2400 X 30% = 7200/ 4 = 180gm/ day. From daily meals /foods - 80gm & rest from good supplement-ENSURE PLUS 30gm per serving with lukewarm water or 100ml milk.
3. Fat (Cook oil) -   2400 X 10% =   240/9 = 27gm/ml

Important Advice.

1. Deep sleep min 8-10 hours at night daily.

2. High-fiber and gas-producing foods can also cause some people to discomfort after gallbladder surgery. So you can consume below foods moderately or some times high like staple foods cereals as much as possible.

3. Daily two-three times additional protein powder from Abbott India named as ENSURE PLUS& start taking 2tsp Aloe vera juice in the morning.

4. Avoid all oily/fried/cream rich or bhaji or junk, salty foods, or outside street foods. Avoid all unhygienic foods—only home-based soft & bland foods which should be low in oil & no or little spices.
5. No packet spices or flavor masalas, salted foods, or cooking salt less than 3 gm per day. No refined sugar or similar raw sugary foods.
6. In Lunch, try to eat Khichdi for 3 days, adding eggs, two white +1 in the evening with snacks.
7. No stress at all. No heavy workout or exercises or activities.
8. Timely food every 2 hours, No meal skipping, 4 main meals breakfast, Lunch, Snacks, Dinner. With 2 -4 times low snacks with fruits, sprouts.
9. Try to consume the right quality foods based on high calories in every snack.
10. Take ENSURE PLUS as a supplement in B.F as well as Bedtime within Lukewarm/Milk.
11. You can consume sweets but max 2 pcs based on straightforward quality Chana, not too much-refined sugar-based sweets or not with high ghee/butter based.
12. No backdated. Old, challan-based foods, mainly vegetables, fruits, fishes.
13. No processed foods, challan, or fridged foods. Always home-based fresh.
14. No smoking & alcohol (although medically prohibited). Sometimes red wine better for cardiac health.

Meal Schedule in a Day (Tentative)

Morning -6/7 am – 300ml freshwater + 1 tsp Honey. Eat 50gm Sprouts duly soaked at last night. After 30 min has Aloe vera Juice.

Break Fast 8 am (Anyone option)– 1) 3-4 pcs. Chapathi /Phulka

OR 50gm rice + mix vegetables,150ml milk. (in case rice separate).

2) 3-4pcs Brown Breads + 1 chana sweet+ 1 -2 egg white + 50gm Curd 15 mins later milk.

3) 4 pcs Idly without chutney but can have sambar or Dahibada same quantity.

4.Oat mals /Porridge/ Dalia 100gm or Dahi Chura + 1 sweet+ 1 Banana

You can also add some regional south Indian breakfast provided almost nil fat/oil & spices & salt. These are always bad for you.

(pl. note: all time, you can add 1-2 egg white, 50gm Chena/yogurt/raita, 150 milk/chana)

10 am – 30gm **Ensure Plus** - with your milk/Lukewarm water

10. 30am_-2 Pcs whole Fruits – 1 citrus +1 other type / sometimes green + fruit salad/

11 am – Veg Soup with papaya, gourds, any type. Added with soya/Nutrela 3-4 days .rest non-veg soup chicken strew 100gm.

Lunch – 12/1 noon – 80 Gm Rice + 2-4 pcs. Roti or 120gm Total-Basmati Rice + 1 serving mix vegetables 100gm Katori + 1 Bowl Dal 30gm (any) + 1 serving soft low oil vegetables 100gm + 50 gm sour curd /Raita .if non-vege. then add 1 pc. fish 100gm fresh quality 3-4 days & 2-3 days chicken strew only without any spices etc., as guided already.

You can eat Paneer/ Cheese up to 100gm slices types/ Chana/Yogurts in the veg case. meals.

Mid Afternoon – 3/4 pm: Fruits, Salad either by whole or dressings.

6 pm – Low-calorie snacks (pick from Breakfast meals) + Green Tea

Dinner – 9.30/10 pm – 50-gm Basmati Rice + 3 pcs Roti + 2 servings of vegetables (1 straight mix and another sprout mixing) OR 120gm best quality basmati rice + 1 serving of paneer 50gm /chana/ curd (do not repeat from other meals). Can alternate if non-veg foods you like Lunch, can add 100gm fresh fish including salmon, tuna, Rohu, chicken apart from the soup can intake 100gm

Bed Time – 10 pm– Supplement ENSURE PLUS 1 scoop with milk 150ml of lukewarm water. (for the first ten days, start this supplement 30gm per serving twice, one after B.F & Next either after evening snacks or at bedtime, later can have three-time B.F/ Eve/ At sleep at night.)

Foods strictly to Avoid

- Foods that are fried, like french fries and potato chips
- High-fat meats, such as bacon, bologna, sausage, ground beef, and ribs. High-fat dairy products, such as cheese, ice cream, cream, whole milk, sour cream, Pizza, and chocolate.
- Foods made with lard or butter.Creamy soups or sauce, Meat gravies.
- Oils such as palm and coconut oil. The skin of chicken or turkey.

Include enough:

- Cereals, Whole-grain slices of bread, Nuts, Seeds, Legumes, Brussels sprouts, Broccoli.

vi) A SAMPLE BALANCED DIET FOR THE PATIENT OF OSTEOARTHRITIS

Age – 53 year, Female, Height – 5.2 ft (157) cm, Weight – 68 kg, BMI – 27.64 (28). Target weight 52 kg, so must reduce 68-52=16 kg (+/- 2kg); Working style- Sedentary-student, Food habits- Non-veg.

Diagnosis – Osteoarthritis, Pre Obesity stage (Asian value)

Targeted weight can be reduced first 2 months 5 kgs; (5X2=10 kg)) Followed by 2 kg/month for 2months (3X2=6 kilograms) can be done if followed proper diet & some yoga/fat burning poses. If you lose weight, then max issues will be solved. More importantly, you have to start maintaining healthy lifestyles by waking 6/7 am and at night bed 11-12 pm max.

(Standard BMI * (for weight) - Range 18.5- 24.9) After > (24-30 overweight , 30> Obesity-I, 35 > Obesity II, 40> obesity III)

Advice – The first target to lose weight 16-18 kg but gradually.

Under Observation for 30 days. Monitor weight on every 7day. Follow up again after 30 days.

1 hour of daily **exercises to come down weight by safe method & retain for future**. (**avoidance** > subject to any injury/ surgery/pregnancy/ knee or joint pain/arthritis/osteoarthritis). Presently to practice at home or home campus only. Supplements all commercial are not safe rather harmful severely.

Recommended Dietary Allowance per day -1400Kcal.

(Ref:1900 kcal/day average sedentary-ICMR-NIN)

1.Carbohydrate – 1400kcal x 50% = 700 kcal/4 = 175gm

2.Protien - 1400kcal x 25% = 350kcal/4 = 88 gm
(preferably veg. protein)

3. Fat -15% -1400kcal X 15% = 210 kcal /9 = 23gm< (cooking oil 2tsf)

4. Antioxidants/Misc – 10 % through vegetables, fruits , liquids etc.

Better to use rice bran oil or Olive oil.

TENTATIVE DIET PLAN (30days-weekly plan)

(Alternatively days, all raw calculation of ingredients)

6.30/7 am – 300ml water + lemon drops/ apple cider vinegar-only 2drops (5ml) + 1 tablespoon CHIA SEEDS (2 hours soaked in same 1 glass water) – drink the total mixture on an empty stomach.

7 am- After 10 min -2 creak cracker biscuit + enough water + 1 cup green tea

7.15am- 8.15 am : Exercises - Then start 15 min yoga poses + Physiotherapy exercises= total 1 hr. *(Avoid : some poses If continuous discomfort & subject to any injury/ surgery/pregnancy/ knee or joint pain/arthritis/osteoarthritis)*

Practice 2-3 times per day @ 30 each time, morning and evening if not fully possible at early morning.

8.30 am Then take 10 min rest & water + green tea/black 1 cup with 1 cream cracker biscuit.

9 am – Breakfast – alternatively (2-3 days)

1) 50gm Plain Oat + fat-free & sugar-free skim milk OR curd 50 gm+1 egg white

2) 2 pc Brown Bread with green salad/1 PC small veg. + 50 gm curd+1 egg white

3) Chira (rice flakes) 30 gm + lemon drops + curd 50 gm + 5 gm raw sugar

During the winter season, use sunlight by this time to get vitamin D

9.30am/10 am - enough water + 1 cup green tea

11 am – 1 guava/apple/green grapes with any citrus fruit like Mosambi. No juices)- (avoid mango, banana, dry fruits all)

12-1 pm –Lunch (**4days /week** non-veg) – 50 gm brown rice (2-3 days/week) OR 2 Phulka roti = 50 gm packet atta (3-4 days /week). + 20 gm Dal (Mug/lentil/urad)+ mix veg (less oil & spices –only homemade) 1 bowl=100 gm + 1 fish rohu-100 gm (simple no curry types). Chicken 1 day/week small leg pc soup form only.

If veg. (3days/week) : 50gm = 2 pcs. plain paneer cream less or 50 gm curd lassi or poppy seeds 20 gm sabzi. *@can add a green salad, sour curd 50gm mandatorily.*

 # Drink water after 30 min of lunch, chew properly during lunch eating.

NO POST LUNCH SLEEP

Tea break ---- if you like, water + 1 cup green tea (if office/ habits).

4 pm – any- 2pcs fruits – 1 guava/1 apple with any citrus fruit like Mosambi. No juices). 11 am and this time- better to have 300 gm whole fruits (as possible).

4-5 pm – some mild walking + freehand exercises - better at park/roof as possible but carefully- avoid going outside from home.; (pollution free zone and maintain physical distance); avoid brisk walking in case of joint pain, etc. as said above) else speed-walking

6/7 pm –evening – Any light calorie meal – 2 pc Idly/ 2 pcs. bread (no butter)/OR, rice flakes/muri 50gm with + green salad; (fast/junk foods)

8 pm - Then green tea & Cream Cracker Biscuit 1-2 pcs.

9.30 pm – Dalia 50gm (3-4 days/week); plain Oat 50m OR 1 pc roti + 20 dal + 100 gm mix veg. + 1 egg white (3-4 days)/ 1 Pc. Small fish

VEG meals mostly all days (5days/week at dinner) : 2-3 pcs. paneer+ 50 gm green salad/Raita can add. No egg/fish in case veg. day.

Always low quantity than Lunch, avoid rice positively. # Avoid fish or chicken at dinner till the next diet plan.

<u>**Some common tips to follow daily strictly.**</u>

Without home exercises or activities like walking at the roof or open areas (keeping social distancing) 1-2kms = 30 in at a time daily + 30 min yoga at floor or bed.–so be serious & start practicing. (subject to any injury/ surgery/pregnancy/ knee or joint pain/arthritis/osteoarthritis).

- Diet and exercises are both mandatory timely as per schedule. Enough calcium with vitamin D from food and natural sources are needed to be better at home rather than medication
- Must have enough water and electrolytes. Min 3 ltr. water/electrolytes

- Best vegetables – all gourds like Lau, parwal, ridge gourd, ash gourd, and capsicum, cucumber, lettuce, drumstick (sajne data). *Avoid potatoes, sweet potatoes, all raw ground level greens.*
- Sleep timely only 7 hours only at 10-5 am/ 11-6am.No post-lunch sleep.
- Avoid: Mustard oil & other seeds based oils (better to use Olive Oil for snacks or rice bran in general use in cooking.)
- Rigorous activities, dynamic lifestyles, timely low-calorie meals can help you only.
- Only brown Rice, if like rice (2-3 days max/week) even you should eat brown rice available. Better add roti max 2-3 pcs per serving or meal to avoid fat. Better dal- Moog, avoid other dal.
- Avoid Soya bean, raw beans, too many sprouts in meals, or raw/soaked. Cow's etc., milk.
- (NO Banana, dry fruits, mango, sweet all juices or same types fruits, all nuts, and dry fruits).
- For skin allergy, avoid dust rust, responsible; check by the tests, no stress, and no overnight work. Stool very clear every day.
- Add salad like cucumber, some onion, capsicum, green boil tomatoes.
- Little more/slightly can add – Garlic, Ginger, some iodized salt but less than 5gm including cooking. Some coastal fishes contain omega 3-6-9 fatty acids rich sources for fair skin, hair, overall anti oxidations.

Avoid completely/ very, very low quantity:

- All beans, soya and soya products, brinjal, all roots/ underground vegetables, spinach, local greens like reddish or pat leaves, etc., all seeds, mostly all sprouts, Ragi, Millet based foods products.

- Oils – All must stop, safe only Olive Oil Or any white oil preferably Rice Bran, Butter, ghee
- No mental stress or anger. Drink more water, electrolytes 300 ml twice a day but without sugar, may add rock salt – Himalaya salt.
- Yoga or Physiotherapy should be practice daily two to three times around 5-6 am (early morning, evening (not mandatory) & 30min after dinner or night meal at 10 pm at bedtime. (after a gentle short walking/wandering at home).
- Females must check timely menstruation (period), maintain proper hygiene also and covid safety. If you lose weight, then you can expect regular menstruation. So keep patience and follow a diet with exercises properly.
  - Yoga or few fat-burning poses should be practiced daily two to three times around 6.30 am (early morning but evening not mandatory) but training at bedtime, only easy poses & 30min after dinner or night meal at 10 pm rest.

Genetical factors: Osteoarthritis can be due to genetic factors.

1. Interleukins
2. VitaminD and its receptors (VDR)
3. Structural proteins related to loss of cartilages
4. Mitochondrial genetics is also responsible.
5. Obesity,
6. Oxidative stress
7. Smoking
8. Estrogen disturbances or other hormones

Disclaimer: All content related to diseases written here is based on general conditions but not for severity or any severe cases, .i.e. person to person variable. The Author is not responsible for any circumstances.

Note:

vii) A SAMPLE BALANCED DIET FOR THE PATIENT OF POLYCYSTIC OVARIAN DISEASE

Age - 27 year, Female, Height-5.2ft. =157 cm, Weight – 64 kg, BMI = 26.02 (26); [Standard BMI * (for weight) - Range 18.5-22.9); 23-25=Over weight; After > 24-30 =pre obesity, 30-40 = Obesity I> obesity II and 50 above Obesity III].   Target weight = 54 (+/-2) kg;

Working style- student (Sedentary) - Non-veg.

Diagnosis – pre-Obesity stage (Asian value), PCOD, excess body fat/bulky, Hyper Prolactinemia.

The target weight should be 54kg, so you need to lose 64-54=10 kg gradually. Targeted weight can be reduced first 2months @ 3 kg. =6kg. Followed by 2 kgX2months can be done (tentative plan) if followed proper diet & some yoga/fat burning poses, freehand, walking.

<u>Advice</u> – The first target to lose weight 10-12 kg but gradually. Under observation for 30 days. Monitor weight on every 7day.

<u>Daily Calorie Requirement – 1400kcal/day by foods</u>
(Ref:1900 kcal/day average sedentary-ICMR-NIN)

1 hour of daily exercises to come down weight by safe method & retain for future (avoidance > *subject to any injury/ surgery/pregnancy/ knee or joint pain/arthritis/osteoarthritis). Presently to practice at home or home campus only. Supplements all commercial are not safe rather harmful severely.*

<u>Recommended Dietary Allowance/ day-</u>
<u>Net Energy 1400Kcal (+/-100kcal)</u>

1.Carbohydrate – 1400kcal x 50% = 700 kcal/4 = 175gm

2.Protien - 1400kcal x 30% = 420kcal/4 = 105 gm (preferably veg. protein good.)

3.Fat -15% -1400kcal X 15% = 210 kcal /9 = 23gm< (only cooking oil 2.5tsf)

4.Antioxidants/Misc - 5% through additional vegetables, fruits, electrolytes etc.

Better to use edible Olive oil could be the best.

TENTATIVE DIET PLAN (for the 30days-weekly plan)

(Alternatively days, all raw calculation of ingredients)

6.30 am – Wake up and After refreshments; 300ml water + 2 tablespoon CHIA SEEDS raw black (2 hours soaked in same 1 glass water or make dust) + 2 tbsp Aloe vera Juice (Dabur/Apollo co.) and make a total mixture as detox water at empty stomach after brushing. (Raw Chia seeds available online aprx. 200/- costs and ACV any brands).

6.45 am- water + 2 pc cream cracker biscuit + Black tea 1 cup

Exercises-7.30 am -8 am: 15 Min Yoga poses as pic provided + 15 min freehand + 30 min morning walking at the safe zone. Gradually increase to speed. (Avoid: If continuous discomfort & subject to any injury/ surgery/pregnancy/ knee or joint pain/arthritis/osteoarthritis. If discontinued, you cannot expect quick results/ if initially feeling discomfort may practice 3-4 times splitting ways.). Practice 2-3 times per day @ 30 in each time, morning and evening.

8.30 am- Then take 10 min rest & water + green tea/black tea/Green Coffee 1 cup with 2 cream cracker biscuit. No coffee. (tea biscuit any 1-2 time in the morning)

9am-Breakfast-alternatively.(2-days-each)

40gm Plain Oat + mix vegetables 50 gm +1 egg white (2-3 days/week)

4) 1 pc roasted Brown Bread with green salad/1 PC small veg. Sandwich + 50 gm curd + 1 egg white (1-2days/week).
5) 30 gm Poha/Upma added with mix vegetables 50 gm + 1 egg white. (1-2days/week).
6) Sattu sharbat 50 gm added with pink salt 5gm + black pepper [if no acidity-1-2days].

10 am at home – half glass Mosambi/orange Juice or

 whole fruits: 1+1pc guava/apple/berries 10 pcs as per local availability. (No juices- avoid mango, banana, dry fruits, citrus, and juices-all)

1 pm –Lunch (Non-veg : 5days /week non-veg.) – 2pcs=20gm packet Atta roti OR 30 gm brown rice (3 days /week) + 20 gm soupy any dal + mix veg. (less oil & spices- only homemade) 1 bowl=100 gm + 100 gm fish (simple no curry types/no challan or marine fish). Chicken 1 day/week small liver/leg pc. (50 gm). No red meat.

If veg. (2days/week) all green and gourds vegetables 100gm + @ *can add a green salad.50gm +50 gm curd (all in case of veg. recipe)*

Drink water after 30 min of lunch, chew properly during lunch eating.

No Post Lunch Sleep if at home - some home-based walking and sitting work. You can take some sitting rest but not deep sleep.

4 pm – any- 2pcs fruits/Biscuits – 1 guava/1 apple/ 1 biscuit

5 pm-5.30 pm – some mild walking -*avoid going outside from home.; (pollution free zone and maintain physical distance)*

7pm – 30 gm Muri/ dried ready to eat chira + 50 gm green salad/ soaked sprouts

OR 2 pcs Idly + some sambar (No coconut chutney)

8pm-some water 1 pcs Biscuit + 1 cup green tea

Dinner- 9/9.30 pm (preferably veg.) – 2 pcs. Roti = 40gm atta (3days/week) OR Dalia 50gm (3-4 days/week) OR plain Oats 30gm + 20 dal + 100 gm mix veg.

Non-Veg. (4days/week) + 1 pcs =50gm fresh fish without curry OR egg white only. *NO chicken* at dinner. *NO Mutton till further notice.* No curry/gravy/dalna/ Better to have 1 egg/ only fish without curry.

Egg max 2 white per day during snacks. If not fish, then better have veg. Meals.

VEG meals (min. 3days/week): 50gm Mix vegetables with rajma/paneer 2pc=20gm + 50 gm green salad as Raita/curd 50gm can-add.
Always low quantity than lunch, avoid rice positively at dinner. # Avoid chicken at dinner till the next diet plan. Post dinner – 15 min home-based walking if possible and drink water after 15 min both in Lunch cum dinner

By 11 pm - Tight sleep. Early wake-up; late-night work may gain weight or stress.

Some common Tips to follow daily strictly.

- Make a day-wise diet plan as per your family routine, keeping my diet (quantity, recipes, foods items, timing) remains the same. Timely follow-up diet and exercises must.

- Must follow this low-calorie diet, low carbs, no such sugar and salt diet with intense exercises needed. Must avoid all fast foods and junk foods.

- Buy a kitchen weight machine for precise measurements at home.

- Best vegetables – all gourds like Lau, parwal, capsicum, cucumber, lettuce, drumstick (sajne data) add more figs, spinach, and kulekhada leaves Thod, Mocha, broccoli beet, carrot as daily as possible. Avoid potatoes, sweet potatoes, all raw saag. Greens, vegetables, fruits, as guided above, are only helpful for you. Some restrictions are given below

- No fast, junk, saturated, trans-fat-based foods or meals like pizza, burger, Biriyani all types, chowmin. Must STOP all kinds of fried foods like street foods, even home-based no fried foods and no fried vegetables. No cola products, no alcohol, smoking,

- Sleep only 7 hours only at 10-5 am/ 11-6am.No post-lunch sleep. Be dynamic as possible but never be at a place for a long time sitting, rather always movements oriented

- Exercises (as mail) as more possible 1hours preferably early morning for best results.

- Avoid mustard oil & other seeds based oils (better use Olive Oil for snacks or rice bran in general use in cooking.). NO butter, ghee, cheese, all cream rich foods or NO oily or fried foods, bhaji/bhaja, salted, sweeteners /high sugar-based sweets, ice cream, at all. In a word – no fast or junk foods.

- Rigorous activities, dynamic lifestyles, timely low-calorie meals can help you only.

- Check the quantity of brown 50gm< or white Rice 30gm< if like rice. Better dal Moog or arahat dal. Avoid other dal. Avoid excessive Soya bean, raw beans, too many sprouts in meals, or natural/soaked. All fat milk and cream or fat-rich dairy foods also. If the habit of drinking Milk, then may have 1 glass=200 ml pasteurized Milk after dinner just before sleep or post-breakfast 9without fruits/juices that time).
- NO Banana, dry fruits, mango, sweet all juices or same types fruits, all nuts, and hydrated fruits
- Can add salad like cucumber, some onion, capsicum, all vegetables must be cooked properly.
- Drink more water and electrolytes rather than simple sugar-rich foods. Have lemon/orange Glucon –D, avoid lemon water

AVOID in PCOD :

- All SUGAR and salt-rich foods, No cream foods, No challan/backdated fridged foods.
- More importantly, if you can lose weight, then the PCOD issue may be solved. Try to start exercises gradually.
- All brinjal, all roots/ underground vegetables, spinach, local greens like reddish or pat leaves, etc., all seeds, mostly all sprouts, Ragi, Millet based foods products. All marine fishes to avoid.
- Oils – All must stop, safe only Olive Oil Or any white oil preferably Rice Bran, Butter, ghee
- Little more/slightly can add – Garlic, Ginger, some iodized salt but less than 5gm including cooking. Some coastal fishes contain omega 3-6-9 fatty acids rich sources for fair skin, hair, overall anti oxidations.
- No mental stress or anger. Drink more water, electrolytes 300 ml twice a day but without sugar, may add rock salt – Himalaya salt.

- Check timely menstruation (period), maintain proper hygiene also and covid safety. If you lose weight, then you can expect regular menstruation. So keep patience and follow a diet with exercises properly.
  - Yoga or few fat-burning poses should be practice daily two to three times around 6.30 am (early morning. evening (not mandatory) but training at bedtime, only easy poses & 30min after dinner or night meal at 10 pm at rest. (after a gentle short walking/wandering at home just after Yoga poses)

Disclaimer: All content related to diseases written here is based on general conditions but not for severity or any severe cases, .i.e. person to person variable. The Author is not responsible for any circumstances.

Note

*

*

*

*

*

*

*

*

*

*

21. BIBLIOGRAPHY

1.   https://www.who.int/news-room/fact-sheets/detail/obesity-and-overweight.

2.   Romieu, I., Dossus, L., Barquera, S., Blottière, H. M., Franks, P. W., Gunter, M., Hwalla, N., Hursting, S. D., Leitzmann, M., Margetts, B., Nishida, C., Potischman, N., Seidell, J., Stepien, M., Wang, Y., Westerterp, K., Winichagoon, P., Wiseman, M., Willett, W. C., & IARC working group on Energy Balance and Obesity (2017). Energy balance and obesity: what are the main drivers?. Cancer causes & control: CCC, 28(3), 247–258.https://doi.org/10.1007/s10552-017-0869

3.   https://www.who.int/cardiovascular_diseases/global-hearts/Global_hearts_initiative/en/

4.   https://www.who.int/health-topics/cardiovascular-diseases/

5.   Reddy, K. S., & Katan, M. B. (2004). Diet, nutrition, and the prevention of hypertension and cardiovascular diseases. Public Health Nutrition, 7(1a), 167–186. http://doi.org/10.1079/PHN2003587

6.   Bhupathiraju, S. N., & Tucker, K. L. (2011). Coronary heart disease prevention: nutrients, foods, and dietary patterns. Clinica Chimica Acta; international journal of clinical chemistry, 412(17-18), 1493–1514. https://doi.org/10.1016/j.cca.2011.04.038

7.   Graham, I., Cooney, M., Bradley, D. et al. Dyslipidemias in the Prevention of Cardiovascular Disease: Risks and Causality. Curr Cardiol Rep 14, 709–720 (2012). https://doi.org/10.1007/s11886-012-0313-7

8.   Lee Y, Siddiqui WJ. Cholesterol Levels. [Updated 2019 Jun 3]. In: StatPearls [Internet]. Treasure Island (FL): StatPearls Publishing; 2020 Jan-. Available from: https://www.ncbi.nlm.nih.gov/books/NBK542294/#

9.   https://www.who.int/gho/ncd/risk_factors/cholesterol_text/en/

10. Halpern, A., Mancini, M. C., Magalhães, M. E., Fisberg, M., Radominski, R., Bertolami, M. C., Bertolami, A., de Melo, M. E., Zanella, M. T., Queiroz, M. S., & Nery, M. (2010). Metabolic syndrome, dyslipidemia, hypertension, and type 2 diabetes in youth: from diagnosis to treatment. Diabetology & metabolic syndrome, 2, 55. https://doi.org/10.1186/1758-5996-2-55

11. Wilcox, G. (2005). Insulin and insulin resistance. The Clinical biochemist. Reviews, 26(2), 19–39.

12. American Diabetes Association Diabetes Care 2019 Jan; 42(Supplement 1): S13-S28.https://doi.org/10.2337/dc19-S002

13. Carlsund, Å., & Söderberg, S. (2018). Living with type 1 diabetes as experienced by young adults. Nursing Open, 6(2), 418–425. https://doi.org/10.1002/nop2.222

14. Wu, Y., Ding, Y., Tanaka, Y., & Zhang, W. (2014). Risk factors contributing to type 2 diabetes and recent advances in treatment and prevention. International journal of medical sciences, 11(11), 1185–1200. https://doi.org/10.7150/ijms.10001

15. https://www.who.int/news-room/fact-sheets/detail/diabetes

16. Yau M, Maclaren NK, Sperling M. Etiology and Pathogenesis of Diabetes Mellitus in Children and Adolescents. [Updated 2018 Feb 13]. In: Feingold KR, Anawalt B, Boyce A, et al., editors. Endotext [Internet]. South Dartmouth (MA): MDText.com, Inc.; 2000-. https://www.ncbi.nlm.nih.gov/books/NBK498653/

17. Korsgren, S., Molin, Y., Salmela, K., Lundgren, T., Melhus, A., & Korsgren, O. (2012). On the etiology of type 1 diabetes: a new animal model signifying a decisive role for bacteria eliciting an adverse innate immunity response. The American journal of pathology, 181(5),1735–1748. https://doi.org/10.1016/j.ajpath.2012.07.022

18. Cantley, J., & Ashcroft, F. M. (2015). Q&A: insulin secretion and type 2 diabetes: why do β-cells fail?. BMC biology, 13, 33. https://doi.org/10.1186/s12915-015-0140-6

19. Abourawi F. I. (2006). Diabetes mellitus and pregnancy. The Libyan journal of medicine, 1(1), 28–41. https://doi.org/10.4176/060617

20. Asif, M. (2014). The prevention and control of type-2 diabetes by changing lifestyle and dietary patterns. Journal of education and health promotion, 3, 1. https://doi.org/10.4103/2277-9531.127541

21. https://www.who.int/health-topics/hypertension/#tab=tab_1

22. Dua, S., Bhuker, M., Sharma, P., Dhall, M., & Kapoor, S. (2014). Body mass index relates to blood pressure among adults. North American Journal of medical sciences, 6(2), 89–95. https://doi.org/10.4103/1947-2714.127751

23. Banerjee, S. (2020). The Essence of Indian Indigenous Knowledge in the perspective of Ayurveda, Nutrition, and Yoga. *Research & Reviews in Biotechnology & Biosciences*, 7(2), 20–27. http://www.biotechjournal.in/issues.php?yid=20&vid=45.

24. Singh, S., Shankar, R., & Singh, G. P. (2017). Prevalence and Associated Risk Factors of Hypertension: A Cross-Sectional Study in Urban Varanasi. International journal of hypertension, 2017, 5491838, https://doi.org/10.1155/2017/5491838

25. http://origin.searo.who.int/topics/hypertension/en/

26. Raghvendra K. Dubey, Suzanne Oparil, Bruno Imthurn, Edwin K. Jackson Cardiovascular Research, Volume 53, Issue 3, February 2002, Pages 688 708, https://doi.org/10.1016/S0008-6363(01)00527-2

27. Manrique, C., Lastra, G., Gardner, M., & Sowers, J. R. (2009). The renin-angiotensin-aldosterone system in hypertension: roles of insulin resistance and oxidative stress. The Medical clinics of North America, 93(3), 569–582. https://doi.org/10.1016/j.mcna.2009.02.014

28. Re R. N. (2009). Obesity-related hypertension. The Ochsner Journal, 9(3), 133–136.

29. Bazzano, L. A., Green, T., Harrison, T. N., & Reynolds, K. (2013). Dietary approaches to prevent hypertension. Current

hypertension reports, 15(6), 694–702. https://doi.org/10.1007/s11906-013-0390-z

30. Steinberg, D., Bennett, G. G., & Svetkey, L. (2017). The DASH Diet, 20 Years Later. JAMA, 317(15), 1529–1530. https://doi.org/10.1001/jama.2017.1628.

31. Misciagna G, Centonze S, Leoci C, Guerra V, Cisternino AM, Ceo R, et al. Diet, physical activity, and gallstones are a population-based case-control study in southern Italy. Am J Clin Nutr. 1999;69(1):120–126.

32. Compagnucci AB, Perroud HA, Batalles SM, Villavicencio R, Brasca A, Berli D, et al. A nested case-control study on dietary fat consumption and its risk gallstone disease. J Hum Nutr Diet. 2016;29(3):338–344. DOI: 10.1111/jhn.12332.

33. Tsai CJ, Leitzmann MF, Willett WC, Giovannucci EL. Fruit and vegetable consumption and risk of cholecystectomy in women. Am J Med. 2006;119(9):760–767. DOI: 10.1016/j.amjmed.2006.02.040.

34. Nordenvall C, Oskarsson V, Wolk A. Fruit, and vegetable consumption, and cholecystectomy risk: a prospective cohort study of women and men. Eur J Nutr. 2016. doi:10.1007/s00394-016-1298-6.

35. Kameda H, Ishihara F, Shibata K, Tsukie E. Clinical and nutritional study on gallstone disease in Japan. Jpn J Med. 1984;23(2):109–113.

36. Tsai CJ, Leitzmann MF, Willett WC, Giovannucci EL. Long-term intake of dietary fiber and decreased risk of cholecystectomy in women. Am J Gastroenterol. 2004;99(7):1364–1370. DOI: 10.1111/j.1572-0241.2004.30153.x.

37. Jorgensen T, Jorgensen LM. Gallstones and diet in a Danish population. Scand J Gastroenterol. 1989;24(7):821–826. DOI: 10.3109/00365528909089221

38. Davidovic DB, Tomic DV, Jorg JB. Dietary habits as a risk factor of gallstone disease in Serbia. Acta Chir Iugosl. 2011;58(4):41–44. DOI: 10.2298/ACI1104041D.

39. Shin Y, Choi D, Lee KG, Choi HS, Park Y. Association between dietary intake and post laparoscopic cholecystectomy symptoms in patients with gallbladder disease. Korean J Intern Med. 2017.

40. Koeth RA, Wang Z, Levison BS, Buffa JA, Org E, Sheehy BT, et al. Intestinal microbiota metabolism of L-carnitine, a nutrient in red meat, promotes atherosclerosis. Nat Med. 2013;19(5):576–585. DOI: 10.1038/nm.3145.

41. Tsai CJ, Leitzmann MF, Willett WC, Giovannucci EL. Long-term intake of trans-fatty acids and risk of gallstone disease in men. Arch Intern Med. 2005;165(9):1011–1015. DOI: 10.1001/archinte.165.9.1011

42. Moerman CJ, Smeets FW, Kromhout D. Dietary risk factors for clinically diagnosed gallstones in middle-aged men. A 25-year follow-up study (the Zutphen study) Ann Epidemiol. 1994;4(3):248–254. DOI: 10.1016/1047-2797(94)90104-X.

43. Caroli-Bosc FX, Deveau C, Peten EP, Delabre B, Zanaldi H, Hebuterne X, et al. Cholelithiasis and dietary risk factors: an epidemiologic investigation in Vidauban, Southeast France. General Practitioner's group of Vidauban. Dig Dis Sci. 1998;43(9):2131–2137. DOI: 10.1023/A:1018879819301.

44. Jessri M, Rashidkhani B. Dietary patterns and risk of gallbladder disease: a hospital-based case-control study in adult women. J Health Popul Nutr. 2015;33(1):39–49.

45. Tseng M, DeVellis RF, Maurer KR, Khare M, Kohlmeier L, Everhart JE, et al. Food intake patterns and gallbladder disease in Mexican Americans. Public Health Nutr. 2000;3(2):233–243. DOI: 10.1017/S1368980000000276.

46. Conter RL, Roslyn JJ, Pitt HA, DenBesten L. Carbohydrate diet-induced calcium bilirubinate sludge and pigment gallstones in the prairie dog. J Surg Res. 1986;40(6):580–587. DOI: 10.1016/0022-4804(86)90101-0.

47. Lee YC, Song DK, Kim JS, Choi CS. Effect of cholestyramine on the formation of pigment gallstone in high carbohydrate diet-fed hamsters. J Korean Med Sci. 1996;11(5):397–401. DOI: 10.3346/jkms.1996.11.5.397.

48. Park YH, Park SJ, Jang JY, Ahn YJ, Park YC, Yoon YB, et al. Changing gallstone disease patterns in Korea. World J Surg. 2004;28(2):206–210. DOI: 10.1007/s00268-003-6879-x.

49. Hauner H. Secretory factors from human adipose tissue and their functional role. Proc Nutr Soc. 2005;64:163–9.

50. Brosseau L, Wells GA, Tugwell P, Egan M, Dubouloz CJ, Casimiro L, Bugnariu N, Welch VA, De Angelis G, Francoeur L, Milne S, Loew L, McEwan J, Messier SP, Doucet E, Kenny GP, Prud'homme D, Lineker S, Bell M, Poitras S, Li JX, Finestone HM, Laferrière L, Haines-Wangda A, Russell-Doreleyers M, Lambert K, Marshall AD, Cartizzone M, Teav A. Ottawa Panel. Ottawa Panel evidence-based clinical practice guidelines for the management of osteoarthritis in adults who are obese or overweight. Phys Ther. 2011;91:843–61.

51. Masuko K, Murata M, Suematsu N, Okamoto K, Yudoh K, Nakamura H, Kato T. A metabolic aspect of osteoarthritis: lipid as a possible contributor to the pathogenesis of cartilage degradation. Clin Exp Rheumatol. 2009;27:347–53.

52. Baker KR, Matthan NR, Lichtenstein AH, Niu J, Guermazi A, Roemer F, Grainger A, Nevitt MC, Clancy M, Lewis CE, Torner JC, Felson DT. Association of plasma n-6 and n-3 polyunsaturated fatty acids with synovitis in the knee: the MOST study. Osteoarthritis Cartilage. 2012;20:382–7.

53. Stürmer T, Sun Y, Sauerland S, Zeissig I, Günther KP, Puhl W, Brenner H. Serum cholesterol and osteoarthritis. The baseline examination of the Ulm Osteoarthritis Study. J Rheumatol. 1998;25:1827–32.

54. Cao Y, Winzenberg T, Nguo K, Lin J, Jones G, Ding C. Association between serum levels of 25-hydroxyvitamin D and osteoarthritis: a systematic review. Rheumatology (Oxford) 2013;52:1323–34.

55. Tong PC, Lee ZS, Sea MM, Chow CC, Ko GT, Chan WB, et al. The effect of orlistat-induced weight loss, without concomitant hypocaloric diet, cardiovascular risk factors and insulin sensitivity in young obese Chinese subjects with or without type 2 diabetes. Arch Intern Med. 2002;162:2428–35.

56. Kelley DE, Kuller LH, McKolanis TM, Harper P, Mancino J, Kalhan S. Effects of moderate weight loss and orlistat on insulin resistance, regional adiposity, and fatty acids type 2 diabetes. Diabetes Care. 2004;27:33–40.

57. Parillo M, Rivellese AA, Ciardullo AV, Capaldo B, Giacco A, Genovese S, et al. A high-monounsaturated-fat/low-carbohydrate diet improves peripheral insulin sensitivity in non-insulin-dependent-diabetic-patients. Metabolism. 1992;41(12):1373–8.

58. Banerjee, S. (2020). Implementation of the vegan diet among obese hypothyroid housewives living in metro cities - A review. International Research Journal of Medical Sciences, 8(1), 21–24.

59. Triggiani V, Tafaro E, Giagulli VA, Sabbà C, Resta F, Licchelli B, et al. Role of iodine, selenium, and other micronutrients in thyroid function and disorders. Endocr Metab Immune Disord Drug Targets 2009;9:277-94.

60. Srivastav A, Maisnam I, Dutta D, Ghosh S, Mukhopadhyay S, Chowdhury S. Cretinism revisited. Indian J Endocrinol Metab 2012;16(Suppl 2): S336-7.

61. Franceschi S, Levi F, Negri E, Fassina A, La Vecchia C. Diet, and thyroid cancer: A pooled analysis of four European case-control studies. Int J Cancer 1991;48:395-8.

62. Leung AM, Pearce EN, Braverman LE. Perchlorate, iodine, and the thyroid. Best Pract Res Clin Endocrinol Metab 2010;24:133-41

63. Banerjee, S. (2018). A Study on Relationship between Hypothyroidism and Non-Alcoholic Fatty Liver Disease among Obese Women in Kolkata Intervening with Diet. International Journal of Research and Development, 3(10), 43–48.

64. Banerjee, S. (2019). Study on Yoga Intervention along with Diet on Hypothyroidism Associated with Obesity among Sedentary Working Women in West Bengal. International Journal of Yoga and Allied Sciences, 8(1), 2278–5159.

65. Meireles, D., Gomes, J., Lopes, L. et al. A review of properties, nutritional and pharmaceutical applications of Moringa oleifera: integrative approach on conventional and traditional Asian medicine. ADV TRADIT MED (ADTM) 20, 495–515 (2020). https://doi.org/10.1007/s13596-020-00468-0

66. www.1mg.com; Retrieved on 15th Dec 2021

67. www.abbott.com; Nutrition information. Retrieved 15th Dec 20

68. Banerjee, S. (2020). Uses of technologies & social media for diet and exercise awareness among obese, hypothyroid, and pre-diabetic women – A case study in West Bengal. Journal of

Xi'an University of Architecture & Technology, 12(3), 4682–4688. https://doi.org/https://doi.org/10.37896/JXAT12.03/426

69. https://www.european.review.org

70. Banerjee, S., Srivastava, S., & Giri, A. K. (2020). Possible nutritional approach to cope up COVID-19 in Indian perspective. Advance Research Journal of Medical and Clinical Science, 06(06), 207–219.

71. Banerjee, S., & Samaddar, B. (n.d.). Impact of COVID-19 Lockdown on Overweight Typically Managed by easy diet Planning-A Mini-Review (Vol. 10). www.ijtonline.com

72. http://www.dietdoctor.com.

73. Pandey, M. M., Rastogi, S., & Rawat, A. K. S. (2013). Indian Traditional Ayurvedic System of Medicine and Nutritional Supplementation. Evidence-Based Complementary and Alternative Medicine, 2013, 376327. https://doi.org/10.1155/2013/376327

74. Cucinotta, D., & Vanelli, M. (2020). WHO declares COVID-19 a pandemic. Acta Biomedica, 91(1), 157–160. https://doi.org/10.23750/abm.v91i1.9397

75. WHO. (2017). Maternal, newborn, child, and adolescent health. Global Strategy for Infant and Young Child Feeding, August, 1–30.

76. Banerjee, S. (2020). Reconsideration of eating time of citrus and fibrous fruits to assure maximum health benefits by proper nutrition: Empirical vs. Theoretical. Food and Scientific Reports, 1(November), 58–67.

77. Banerjee, S., & Samaddar, B. (n.d.). Impact of COVID-19 Lockdown on Overweight Typically Managed by easy diet Planning-A Mini-Review. 10, 1. www.ijtonline.com

78. Naja, F., & Hamadeh, R. (2020). Nutrition amid the COVID-19 pandemic: a multi-level framework for action. European

Journal of Clinical Nutrition. https://doi.org/10.1038/s41430-020-0634-3.

79. Banerjee, S. (2020, December). Nutrition Facts, Health Benefits and Aggregate Nutrient Density Index (ANDI) of Roots and Tubers Vegetables. *Agriculture & Food*, 2(12), 588–590.

80. Emergency, P. H., Concern, I., & Health, M. (2020). Mental health and psychosocial considerations during the COVID-19 outbreak. March, 1–6.

81. Banerjee, S., & Ghosh, J. (2019). Psychological Disorders & Nutrition: A handbook on diet and nutrition for mental health (Kindle (ed.); 1st ed.). Amazon. https://www.amazon.in.

82. Banerjee, S. (2020). Interactions between common foods and drugs - a narrative review. Asian Journal of Pharmaceutical Research, 10(3), 188. https://doi.org/10.5958/2231-5691.2020.00033.7

*** ***